self

self

Dr Linda Friedland

First published in 2005 by

Tafelberg Publishers
Heerengracht 40, Cape Town 8000
Registration nr.: 51/02378/06

10 9 8 7 6 5 4 3 2 1

Publisher Anita Pyke
Editor Glynn Newlands
Design Valerie Phipps-Smith
Cover design Petal Palmer
Illustrations Izak Vollgraaf
Index Cecily van Gend

Printed and bound by Paarl Print, Oosterland Street,
Paarl, South Africa

ISBN 0 624 04286 3

For Peter

Contents

Acknowledgements

My heartfelt thanks to my loving parents, Julie and Boomie, and my family, who gave me the opportunity to pursue the study of medicine but also to shape and develop so many ideas beyond science. Your support and love to the entire clan has allowed me to do so much. To Selma, for the encouragement and literary guidance each step of the way.

To my many profound teachers – my patients. I thank those who allowed me to share their stories with you especially Professor Jeanne Zaidel Rudolph. To the many inspiring women and special friends in my life who constantly challenge and shape my fascination and passion for women's life and health issues.

To Rachel and Elizabeth, who maintain equilibrium in the tumult of life.

To Anita Pyke, my remarkable publisher at Tafelberg, for her constant guidance, direction and sharp intelligence. She remained a steadfast beacon of light through some very long days, weeks and months. To Glynne Newlands for her comprehensive editing and also for prodding me to achieve greater clarity. And also to Janita Holzhausen for her assistance and guidance in the final stages.

To Roni Witkin in London, my mentor, who truly provided the impetus for me to complete this book finally. I deeply appreciate such insight, clarity and constant professional guidance.

To my husband, Peter, who has given me the wings to fly and keeps me grounded at the same time. This book could not have been written without his wisdom, vision and love. I owe more than gratitude to the genuine blessings in my life – Gavriel, Leora, Yael, Aaron and Benjamin.

Linda Friedland

Introduction

I believe that a book is a profound meeting place between an author and the reader. You as the reader bring almost as much energy and creativity to this book as I do. By using it to enhance your life, you give it wings!

In the writing of this book, my wish is to simply transmit information and knowledge clearly, responsibly and in an inspiring way to encourage you to improve yourSELF. You have the power to take charge of your life path and your personal health.

SELF is about the healing, unfolding, growing and accepting of your unique life. It encourages you to truly take care of yourSELF, optimise your health, celebrate your life, make peace with your body, indulge your interests and passions, enjoy emotional wellbeing and begin to nurture yourSELF.

Although you live in the information age, there is much confusion about which 'truth' to believe. Women of all ages are suffering from many devastating illnesses, and they are more depressed, fatigued and discontent than ever before. Even well women feel less than healthy and in the midst of this e-age, where technology should have freed you up, you may feel overloaded, stressed and at risk for ill-health.

SELF attempts to slice through much of the hype and share with you health information which is both responsible and new. There is no point for me as a doctor to hold on to all this knowledge! My duty and my utter joy is to hand it over to you in a motivating way. My intention is to empower you to take charge of your health and your life, to make informed decisions and choices, and to achieve a shift in your lifestyle that is meaningful and energised.

Although the information and principles are relevant to women every-where, I have written this directly to you as a South African woman with all the experiences and complexities of living in this exciting and challenging country.

I also believe that women's health is so much more than women or health. Women's health affects not only your unique body but is central to your family's and community's wellbeing. Women are the primary decision makers in all healthcare.

Health, too, is more than the absence of disease. It is about your quality of living, and this book guides you to take charge of your life, take excellent care of yourSELF and instructs you exactly how to take action to towards a vibrant and healthy SELF.

Dr Linda Friedland

CHAPTER 1

Empower

Introduction

This first chapter is about the incredible freedom you can exercise within your life, to take responsibility for your personal health, to be empowered. Notwithstanding your circumstances or your current state of health, there is always vast energy and healing at your disposal. You do have choices and the ability to administer excellent self-care.

To be empowered is to have a sense of strength and personal control within. More importantly, it means taking full responsibility for your life and no longer blaming others or circumstances for your situation. You may be discontent, overweight or have a serious illness. You may simply want to perk up your health or ensure that you age well. Whatever your situation, you are the driver of your journey and although there are obstacles to confront, there is so much within your grasp. You have the power to make a rational decision to take charge of your life.

Through the process of becoming empowered and taking charge, your health will be enhanced in so many ways. A new world view (how you perceive your world) will be opened up to you as you examine your core beliefs and choose positive lifestyle behaviours. You will learn to create time for yourself, take control of your relationships, and understand and appreciate your body. Your understanding of your emotional and mental self, as well as the concept of total healing, will also deepen. Through reading this chapter, you will begin to appreciate the value of preventive care and get to know your own personal health parameters, possible risk factors for illness, and learn what health screening is required for your particular stage of life.

Empower Quiz
Are you taking charge of your health and your life?

1. Do you exercise for half an hour or more at least three days a week?	Yes/No
2. Do you have a yearly pelvic exam and Pap smear?	Yes/No
3. Do you perform a monthly breast self-exam? (and a yearly mammogram if over 40?)	Yes/No
4. Are you a non-smoker? (or if you have been a smoker, have you quit?)	Yes/No
5. Do you practice safe sex with any new partner?	Yes/No
6. Do you substitute complex carbohydrates (whole grains, fruit and vegetables) for simple ones such as white bread, potatoes and white rice?	Yes/No
7. Do you take a multivitamin every day?	Yes/No
8. Do you consume at least two servings of dairy products or foods fortified with calcium (like orange juice or cereals) each day or take a calcium supplement?	Yes/No
9. Do you keep your alcohol and caffeine intake low?	Yes/No
10. Do you limit your sun exposure?	Yes/No
11. Do you make sure that you understand the results of your lab tests (like Pap smears or biopsies)?	Yes/No
12. Have you explored your family's medical history to look for clues to your genetic or medical risk factors?	Yes/No
13. Do you continuously try to do too much, organising every last minute of your time and feel most often like you are on a roller coaster?	Yes/No
14. Have you established de-stressing routines such as relaxation baths, meditation, reading and other pleasurable activities?	Yes/No
15. Would you/do you seek help if stress or depression becomes unmanageable?	Yes/No
16. Do you allow yourself leisure time and cultivate interests outside of your work and home?	Yes/No
17. Do you express and experience healthy sexuality?	Yes/No

Score yourself:
Give yourself two points for every YES answer and 0 for every NO, for all questions except question 13, where you should give yourself 0 for yes and two points for NO.

26-34 *You have very healthy habits*
Keep doing what you're doing – you generally know how to take care of yourself. You've taken stock of what's important to you and tried to carve out a space in your life for yourself. Continue to take care of yourself by maintaining and enhancing your exercise programme, keep your caffeine and alcohol intake low, limit your sun exposure, eat fewer calories as you age, take a daily multivitamin, go for health screening, participate in meaningful activities and seek help from your doctor or others when you need it.

10-24 *Take charge and see the difference*
Although you are attending to some of your health needs, many important aspects are being neglected in your life. Starting now, discover more ways to become even healthier by taking charge and enhancing your wellbeing. You have the power to make a difference to your energy, your long-term risk of disease, your emotional and mental health. Begin now by following the guidelines in the Health Action Plan laid out for you at the end of this chapter. Seek help from your doctor when necessary, go for essential health screenings, exercise, rest, eat well, stay out the sun, take supplements, find time for yourself and diffuse your stress.

0-10 *You have plenty of room for improvement*
You are not focusing on your health very much, and may be putting your wellbeing at risk. You also do not have very good lifestyle habits. The capacity to take responsibility for your health and your whole life is in your hands. You have a choice right now. Begin by following the Health Action Plan outlined at the end of this chapter. You will not only ensure much better long-term health and ageing, but you will also feel the difference in every area of your life, from your energy to your peace of mind.

You will also minimise your risk of serious illness. Seek help from professionals if need be, go for necessary health screenings, exercise, rest, eat well, find time for yourself and learn how to diffuse your stress.

Jeanne's story

You may perceive Jeanne's story as a miracle or you may choose to see it as a powerful self-healing experience.

Jeanne, the first and only woman to have obtained a Doctorate in Music Composition in South Africa, is the Professor of Music at the University of the Witwatersrand in Johannesburg, and a world-renowned composer, lecturer and performer. She has recently received the Ikhamanga award (highest order possible) by President Thabo Mbeki for her outstanding contribution to the country. She has been commissioned to compose works as illustrious as *He walked to freedom* in honour of Nelson Mandela, and also composed part of the South African national anthem. Her works are performed throughout the world.

Juggling the responsibility of raising five daughters and running a home with a high-powered, competitive career led to chronic exhaustion. Jeanne found herself on a treadmill of frenetic activity; she admits that she was wishing (albeit subconsciously) to be rescued from overwhelming pressure and anguish. She promised herself that on completion of the *Oratoria* for the 1996 Atlanta Games, she would take a rest. She had no idea that this would take the form of a hospital admission, the very day after completion of this piece.

The diagnosis, she says, *'appeared to be nothing short of a death sentence'*. She experienced a full range of emotions: fear, anger, confusion, guilt and disbelief, alternating with questions like *'Why me?'* and then *'Why not me?'* in response to the Hodgkin's lymphoma diagnosis. In the early days of her illness she drove herself and others crazy searching for reasons. Was she being punished, what had she done wrong? She describes how she rationalised that God was in control and this terrible affliction must be for the best. She convinced herself that blind acceptance was a way to show faith.

A spiritual advisor encouraged her to change her approach by explaining that she had the power to alter her path and destiny. This gave her an elevated sense of self-empowerment, which she believes is at the core of true healing.

She describes a turning point that occurred when she knew that she had only one freedom: the freedom to choose how she was going to deal with this challenge. She chose to give meaning to every moment. She chose to live with passion and purpose. She chose to attempt positively and actively to overcome her illness in every way possible. Jeanne's response to her illness was an amazing integration of the two opposing elements required for total healing: the power of surrender and at the very same time taking personal responsibility. *'One can choose to carry one's heavy burden alone, whether it is illness or any of life's difficulties. My own sense of complete liberation came when I made a conscious decision to hand over my heavy burden and give over my healing to God. I also decided to do everything in my power to be proactive in my recovery!'*

While receiving chemotherapy for a full nine months, she became involved in her own wellness strategy. She became knowledgeable in all areas of her medical therapy, and questioned and prodded her doctors for information. She shifted her diet to include only the healthiest, freshest foodstuffs as well as vitamin, mineral and antioxidant supplementation. She learnt new healing modalities including imagery, visualisations and deep breathing. Reflexology and aromatherapy were included in her schedule. *'It was with a strange sense of relief that for the first time in my life, I was entitled to rest and pamper myself. What a high price to pay for being allowed to take it easy!'*

She even expanded her mental and spiritual horizons. *'I found an invaluable source of knowledge and comfort in reading and studying books both of a spiritual and medical nature. I understood new concepts such as how humour and intense laughter can restore health and how the mind-body pathways facilitate healing.'*

Jeanne also explains the power in the support and love of family and community that helped in her healing. *'I was overwhelmed by the response to my illness by friends, family and the entire community.'*

Now many years later, free of cancer, Jeanne continues to pace her life by honouring and listening to the rhythms of her body, continuing to feed her soul with study and prayer, allowing support, nurturing the love and humour in her life, nourishing herself with optimal foodstuffs and supplements, exercising moderately and making choices each day to live with passion and meaning.

You do not need to wait for serious illness to catapult you into developing your personal power. The time to take charge of your life and your health is *now*.

(Note: Although you have the capacity to take charge through a serious illness, there is much beyond your control. You need not feel guilty or try too hard to 'self-heal'. Part of the process of healing is about surrendering to that which is beyond your control. In addition, although you would wish for complete cure, not everything can be fixed, but healing can still take place at many different levels.)

My story

Although I have encountered and treated many patients with cancer or HIV/Aids, unlike Jeanne I have not experienced my own life-threatening illness. But I have had some peculiar medical disorders over the past few years that have forced me to take charge and change direction.

Two years after the birth of my youngest child, I developed many strange physical symptoms that did not fit into a clear category. Medical school and clinical practice had not prepared me for this. It began with a 'complicated migraine' that continued into several months of a 'fuzzy head', vague nausea (similar to jet lag), some memory loss, severe headaches, painful muscles and debilitating fatigue.

The results of extensive diagnostic tests and various specialist opinions could not be neatly packed into a medical box. However, I did receive some not quite mainstream diagnoses and suggested causes from medical colleagues, including 'toxic liver overload', a 'mitochondrial-metabolic disorder', chemical sensitivity (in the form of pesticides, industrial substances in the environment etc), the genetic deficiency of an enzyme in the liver, low grade infections, the emotional and physical stress of a pregnancy or quite a few pregnancies (in my case), or any physical and emotional stress. Possibly life (especially if you are a woman!) in the 21st century?

The most important thing for me was how to deal with this. There was certainly no medical treatment plan, no magic bullet available. I needed to 'take charge'. I needed to take charge of what I ate, what medication or supplements I needed, I needed to gain as much information as possible as to what could be done and how to do it. I became vigilant with my diet and I took good nutritional supplements. I temporarily stopped exercising (I was mainly jogging) and then after a few months changed my exercise modality to one of lower impact, more stretching, balance and breath work. I began meditating at least twice a day and frequently used guided imagery and music.

But the most significant change was what I had to do in my internal world. I had to 'surrender' – a difficult task for a high-energy control freak! At the very same time as taking charge, I also needed to let go: to let go of needing to know and understand it all. To let go of my sense of control of knowing exactly how, when and whether I was going to get better. I was forced to be in that limbo state of the unknown. I was forced to rest much more. I had to change the tempo of my life, and it took a few months to get back on track. (It often takes many years to improve such a condition.)

Now, four years on, although most of the time I feel really well, energetic and focused, I still need to listen to my body's cues to maintain equilibrium. I still experience moments when these symptoms reappear and I know that I am out of balance. It may be due to excessive work or extra strain, but often can be most unexpected. It can be for a few days or a week at a time. I know once again that I need to surrender my sense of control and at the same time take charge of my life and my health and my personal power.

The passage to personal empowerment takes many forms. It occurs in your mental awareness, your emotional growth, your spiritual quest and your physical wellbeing. All these factors influence your health. You have an immeasurable strength within you and by acknowledging and nurturing it, you will begin to live with greater health and meaning.

Take charge
Take charge of your own life

To empower yourself simply means to 'take charge'. Get out of the passenger seat and place yourself in the position of the driver. This means taking personal responsibility for every aspect of your life: for your perceptions, your physical body, your self-image, your relationships, your time and especially your health. It means being an active participant in every relationship that is meaningful. It means being responsible for the decisions you make, the steps you take and the consequences of your actions. Moreover, it means being honest enough to change direction if necessary.

Being in the driver's seat does not mean you have the power to be irresponsible. You cannot simply change direction because you have had enough of the scenery. You cannot just walk out of a job or a marriage without soul searching and being proactive. Begin by looking inward to see what role *you* play in your life situation and if there is anything constructive that you can do to alter the pattern. Obviously, there are situations which may be destructive and no longer serve your values and your goals. In these circumstances, after seeking help or assistance to no avail, it may be time to move on.

You may feel totally out of control because of your hardships or illness. You may be going through a difficult period with children, work or finances. Or you may be experiencing the pain of loss, loneliness or depression. You cannot dramatically change your external environment but you certainly can change your internal responses to these situations. Taking responsibility for all aspects of your life means just that. It does not mean you get into a spiral of self-blame and guilt. You do not bring illness or hardship upon yourself. To truly empower yourself demands a conscious decision to take ownership of your life to the best of your ability.

Take charge of your perceptions

To take charge may involve a change in your perceptions and your world view: how you see things, interpret them and then internalise them. Your thoughts, emotions, desires, likes, dislikes, feelings, fears, judgments, prejudices, hopes and aspirations make up your world view. No two people share the same perception of anything. A picture of beauty for you may be unappealing to me. Food that you desire may cause me nausea.

The thoughts and feelings that constantly spin through your mind ('*I like this, I don't like that', 'I am unsure of x, I am happy with y'*) is an internal conversation based on your deepest core beliefs that you hold on to and assume to be true.

The importance of these perceptions is that they affect not only your mind but also your body. They become encoded into your physical self. Your personal views and experiences are processed through your mind and emotions and literally become internalised into the cells of your body. For example, a woman who becomes depressed after being jilted by her lover will demonstrate physiological changes. Her brain's output of neurotransmitters may become depleted, hormone levels drop, her sleep cycle is seriously disturbed, and even her immune function may be affected. This whole biochemical profile may improve dramatically when she gets over the relationship or falls in love again!

You can begin to take charge by opening up to a different world view, one that slowly replaces fear with hope and trust. A world view that incorporates courage and integrity. A world view of perceptions about yourself, your future and your health that is realistic but also affirming and positive. When you see yourself differently, your personal reality is altered at a physiological level. A clear example of this is in your perception of ageing. Your fear of ageing and deep belief that you are meant to get sick and frail as you age may play a role in accelerating your body's decay and your wilting self-image.

Take charge of your body

With all its blemishes and imperfections, your body is a remarkable design of structure and function. It is a complex mix of numerous systems usually working in perfect harmony. Taking charge requires you to take ownership of this body. You need to have the confidence to say '*this is my body*' and '*I make the decisions about it*' whether it is saying *no* to a sexual advance or *yes* to a course of chemotherapy. You are the driver, the owner

9

of your body, and must participate to the utmost in its upkeep and in all decisions regarding your health.

There are two prerequisites for taking charge of your body. The first is an understanding of how your body functions, and the second is a genuine appreciation of your physical being. Your body has conceived and carried new human life (or at least has the potential to). Your body has an immune protective mechanism to ward off the vast majority of hostile elements in the environment. It maintains homeostasis (balance of all its hormones, enzymes, and regulatory mechanisms) while you are getting on with your life. It controls an internal warmth system during the cold months and cools you down during the hotter months. It secretes the exact amounts of substances required for trillions of finely tuned processes occurring all the time. In addition to the brain's control of movement, sensation and organ function, every cell in your body communicates with every other cell through receptors on their surface. Your body is composed of millions of molecules in a state of continual motion. It is always in a state of renewal and repair. Even with an illness or poor functioning in a specific area, just think of all the processes that are working so well!

Take charge of your time

Most of my conversations with patients or women friends regarding stress management or health and wellbeing or exercise end with the same four words 'I have no time'. Taking control of your life means breaking the woman's mantra of 'no time'. Regardless of how busy you are and your particular challenges, you can begin to pace your life. Instead of marching on at an unrelenting speed over which you have no control, you can consciously create a different pace, one over which you have control. You can also stop yearning for the time you don't have and start constructively creating and using the time that you do have.

A useful and practical way to begin taking charge of your time is to create 'white space' in your schedule. You literally need to take your diary or calendar or palm pilot and create blocks of time specifically for yourself where nothing is planned. The only solution to the overwhelming demands of a multi-tasked working woman or busy mother is to schedule time for yourself with the same degree of respect and seriousness that you would schedule an appointment with your doctor. The process is very simple, although the practice takes some getting used to. You take the calendar and formally mark in a few appropriate time slots. You make this appointment with yourself and short of an emergency, you keep it. If you wait for everything to get done at work, at home or with your family before you allow time for yourself, you will never find it. Your schedule is filled up with your commitments and the needs of others. Everyone manages to get a piece of your time – except you. You obviously need to be realistic but I certainly believe that at least one hour or two per week is possible for everyone. You will determine whether shorter slots more frequently or large chunks of time less frequently are better for you.

When I ask women what stresses them most, one of the most frequent answers is that because there is so much to juggle, they usually find themselves running a few minutes late – for a school lift, a soccer match or a board meeting. This is one of my personal struggles. I always wait until the last possible moment to leave and then run late. There is so much to do that I try to squeeze out the last few moments before rushing off to the next task.

This creates an enormous amount of unnecessary stress as you are constantly thinking about how far you are behind schedule and who is waiting for you. You clutch the steering wheel, your pulse is racing, you've skipped a meal so you are a bit dizzy and you chant that second mantra of South African women 'My life is so hectic!' This common problem is so easily managed by giving yourself an extra five to 10 minutes to get to your next destination. Irrespective of where you are heading, plan now to always leave 10 minutes earlier. This demands a conscious decision from you to alter your pattern. Those minutes can make a huge difference to your internal body responses, your adrenalin and your hormones.

I cannot tell you what a difference this strategy makes to my life. Instead of feeling frantic as I scramble at the last minute searching for my son's shoes or my keys, when I take hold of these extra minutes I feel at peace and empowered. The reason is that I am consciously taking charge of my time.

11

One step better than this is trying to sandwich your plans on both sides with five extra minutes on each side. For example, I will try give myself an extra five minutes to get to a meeting and then use another five after the meeting before the next task. In these transitions, you could do a breathing exercise, get a cup of tea or bottle of water, and sit still before leaving for the athletics meeting at school. There are many 'dead spaces' in your day when you could capture a moment for a stretch or a breath.

Although it is not always possible to achieve this, by consciously aiming to structure your commitments in this way you will break the patterns of 'I have no time' and 'my life is so hectic'.

Take charge of your relationships
You may think that how your relationships unfold is dependant largely on others. You may have a boss who breathes down your neck. You partner may be so controlling over the family's affairs or may expect you to do it all. Your children seem to fire requests and show little appreciation. You may feel that you don't have much control in your work environment or even at home. However, it all begins and ends with you.

Don't wait for love and meaning to find you
Even the love or absence thereof in your life depends on you. There are certainly magical stories of people finding their soulmates in the most unexpected circumstances and living blissfully ever after. But most of the time finding the love you need or keeping the love you have requires effort on your part. You need to start with yourself. If you cannot give yourself the love you say you want, you will never find it in the world outside or in your spouse or lover. Begin by being loving towards yourself and then extending beyond yourself in loving kindness to others.

Stop the self-blame
To be empowered in your relationships is to stop being a victim. Take charge of your life, but not in a way that says 'I caused it all'. Put up the appropriate boundaries that honour you. Do not keep silent in the face of verbal or physical abuse: there is no shame in talking out. 'Keep the peace,

don't make waves' is what allows the abuse to continue. Refuse to tolerate bad behaviour from anyone. Women who continue to blame themselves or go along with the secrets become part of the destructive forces of society.

Choose good company
You cannot choose your work colleagues or your family. But you do have enormous control over whom you spend your spare time with, and the people you invite into your home. Your time and energy are extremely precious to you, so choose to build those relationships that are nourishing. I am not suggesting that you make judgments about people or break off friendships that are based on obligation or tradition. Rather, spend time with people who make you feel good about yourself. The people around you have a great influence on your wellbeing.

Become a better listener
When someone genuinely listens to you, you feel valued and understood. When you do not feel listened to, you are left with an empty feeling. Poor listening skills become an invisible habit. It is certainly a weakness of mine. I have to consciously watch myself as I am about to jump in and interrupt someone or give advice. Or I need to be a little more patient and watch that I don't begin thinking of something else before the person I am listening to has finished. You will be amazed at how quickly old issues and problems become resolved if you simply quiet down and become a better listener. Becoming a better listener is not a passive step but rather will go a long way to empowering your relationships.

Keep your word
By saying you will do something – whether for your children or at work – and then failing to deliver, sets up more and more cracks in your connections. By keeping your word, you are trusted and therefore appreciated.

Be self-reliant
In order to maintain healthy relationships with others, you need to be, self-sufficient in many ways. This does not mean you cannot depend on

others to assist you and be there for you. Strong, intimate and loving relationships are essential for your wellbeing, but truly healthy ties thrive on a balance of self-reliance together with dependence.

Do not miss a chance to show appreciation

When your partner feels appreciated and valued, he will want to be more helpful and supportive towards you. This does not mean you need to be subservient. Running a marriage, a household, a joint budget and rearing a family is a partnership that demands huge responsibility. But the way someone responds when he feels appreciated is priceless. Being empowered is not necessarily about receiving: it may be more about giving. Taking charge of relationships means showing respect and appreciation.

Take charge of your personal health

A core belief of the old world view of medicine is that responsibility for your healthcare rests entirely with your doctor. For many reasons this paradigm has shifted enormously over the past 30 years. Now more than ever before, the responsibility is in your hands.

The genes that you have inherited and the 'will of God' will determine to some extent whether you become ill or not. But if you are active in maintaining your health, many illnesses can be prevented, detected early or looked after really well, and further problems can be avoided.

It is up to you to take charge of your health by making the best lifestyle choices, going for screening and early detection, and being proactive with your risk factors for disease.

Lifestyle choices

The role that health plays is not always easy to see and is often something you take for granted until an illness sets in. In your mad rush to be a better mother, wife, partner, daughter, friend, manager or employee, you may unknowingly sacrifice your health in the process.

You may work long hours, while still continuing to take care of everyone at home, all the time worrying about yesterday and anxious about tomorrow. You may eat on the run, rest little, sleep poorly, drink and smoke too much, exercise too little and lack vision, purpose and joy in your life.

You may also feel the constant pressure to look good and be many things to many people. In the frenetic pace of modern living, you may spend much of your day spiritually, mentally and emotionally disconnected. Everyone else's needs are placed before your own and eventually your body takes a beating.

It's never too late to decide to break this pattern and take charge. Whatever your state of health, body shape or age, you can always improve your condition. Just as you take charge of your career, your mothering and your household, so too take hold of your health.

Relationship with your doctor

Taking charge of your personal health does not mean that you do not need your doctor – quite the contrary. It means that both his or her role and yours have changed. You now should aim to develop a relationship that includes collaborating in the pursuit of your good health.

In addition to examining and treating you when you are ill, your doctor should be available to answer your queries and questions as well as give you any relevant information you may require. He or she should also perhaps remind you of your screening tests such as Pap smears and mammograms and do routine yearly checks of your blood pressure and whatever is required at different ages and stages of your life (see below). But it is ultimately up to you to institute lifestyle changes and ensure that you attend to health screenings for yourself and your family.

Taking charge is also having the confidence to consult with your doctor if you feel he or she is not addressing all your needs. Extensive research has demonstrated that patients who have a good and trusting relationship with their doctors get better clinical results. This may be because they are more motivated to take care of themselves, more comfortable seeking help when problems arise and more willing to follow advice and take medication as prescribed.

A healthy doctor-patient relationship can also give consolation when bad news comes. The relationship itself provides an emotional safety net.

As true as this may be, relationships take time and doctors may often find themselves short of this commodity. You, too, need to be reasonable about your expectations and respectful of boundaries. You cannot expect a parent's love from your doctor, but you can expect clinical expertise with information and compassion. Step one in taking charge here is to communicate freely. Educate yourself about your condition and share your information. Do not hold back for fear of being a nuisance, but perhaps plan to book a longer appointment if you have a lot to discuss. A good clinician is eager to teach and learn, and willing to acknowledge the medicine's limits. You and your doctor can become allies in an effort to not only sustain health but also to sustain hope and meaning in more difficult times.

Take charge with knowledge

To take responsibility, especially for your health, requires gaining information, understanding, insight and the clear facts. To stay one step ahead also requires keeping abreast of new ideas and advances. This enables you to make responsible and informed decisions. The capacity to make the correct choices is often related to how informed and knowledgeable you are as a mother, wife, patient, and in the workplace.

With knowledge, you are in a position of strength and thereby empowered to make clearer decisions. It does not matter at what level you completed formal education; you always have the capacity to increase your understanding.

For example, if you suffer from an illness, you need to become an expert on it. Read, search the Internet, ask questions and empower yourself so that you are aware of your options regarding treatment, side effects and possible ways to improve your condition; then you can become a partner with your doctor in the healing process. Dr Bernie Siegel, an American physician and author, calls those patients who are most informed and active in their healing *ECPs* or exceptional patients. He has validated that these patients have the greatest likelihood of wellbeing and of being cured.

The knowledge required to take charge of your health and your life encompasses both your external and internal worlds. The external knowledge is about gaining scientific medical and health data. The internal knowledge is all about you as an individual, a self-knowledge. You are a unique woman and although you share so much in common with other women, your physical, emotional and psychological make-up is distinctive. For example, most people will respond in a specific way to a certain medication, but there are always a few who have a different reaction. Everyone has a daily 24-hour cycle called a circadian rhythm with many predictable fluctuations in hormone secretion, body temperature and sleep control, but there are so many variations. I am energetic in the morning and not at all a night person; you may potter around getting all your work done after dark. You also have your individual family history, risk factors and genetic make-up. The more you know about this the better. Self-knowledge is about understanding your body and understanding what works best for you, e.g. triggers that physically exhaust you and those that may cause depression or pain.

Physical self-knowledge
Understand your body
Truly empowered means to know your body and every aspect of your physical functioning. You can sense when you are beginning to feel depressed, fatigued, unfit or generally unwell and do something about it.

You may only notice your body when it causes you pain and discomfort. You blame it when it lets you down through injury or illness. You chastise it for not being the right shape or size. At best, you ignore it. But your body allows you to experience everything in your life. Here is the chance to make amends! Participate directly by maintaining your health.

Understand healing
You have within you an extraordinary capacity for healing. Your body is designed to restore equilibrium continually; it wants to be in a state of balance (homeostatis) and it contains numerous mechanisms to keep it functioning in this state of harmony. Your body is constantly changing and renewing itself at a cellular level and this is one of the reasons why physical healing can take place.

You are constantly subjected to outside and internal influences, but your body contains so many internal communication systems that most of the time it can restore this sense of balance. For example, if you become dehydrated by not drinking enough in hot weather, the level of sodium will increase in your blood. This will trigger the release of a hormone through a feedback pathway, which in turn causes the sodium level to be normalised. This happens all the time within millions of cells affecting enzymes, hormones and physiological functions. This is your body healing at its basic level. Sometimes a virus or bacteria will disturb this balance by defeating the body's defences and then it takes a little while longer to restore itself.

When you cut yourself and bleed, a cascade of clotting factors comes into play, allowing the bleeding to stop and then within a few days new tissue grows and healing of this cut occurs. You can view this healed scar on your skin surface. The mending of a broken bone is less visible but is truly remarkable. Sometimes your body is even able to heal from cancer. Your body is constantly combating foreign bacteria and viruses as well as early cancer cells through your immune pathways. Stitches to the cut or a plaster cast to hold the bone or chemotherapy all assist while your body itself initiates its internal healing process.

Yes, there are many instances when this healing system is overcome and is unable to combat the infection or the cancer. The process of recovery is much slower and there are certainly times when complete recovery or disappearance of the illness will never be possible. But there is still so much you can do to optimise your condition.

In addition to standard medical care, you can attempt to boost the healing of your body – and aid the flow of 'your river'– by eating the most nourishing of foods, resting and using relaxation and healing techniques such as meditation and guided imagery. None of the above can do any harm and your active participation may very well help drive the physical healing process.

If you are ill, your main aim is to be completely cured. But it is also important to understand that although not everything can be cured, most things can be healed. Healing is much more than only physical healing.

Healing comes from the words 'holy' and 'whole'. To heal is to become a 'whole' human being who has a 'holy' dimension. Healing can still take place at many levels. Through an illness, you may begin to heal emotional pain or a difficult relationship or develop an untapped spiritual dimension.

Emotional/Psychological self-knowledge

Your life becomes simpler when you begin to truly face up to yourself. It is not always comfortable but is certainly good for you. Understanding your own emotions and mindset and what triggers your mood swings, anger and emotional pain is not purely a psychological exercise to improve your relationships and ease your internal tension. It improves your health.

Viewed through the lens of 21st-century science, anxiety, alienation and hopelessness are not just feelings. Neither are love, serenity and optimism. They are all physiological states that affect your health as clearly as obesity or physical fitness. The brain is the source of these emotional states and then is the gateway to all the organs of your body – to your heart and blood vessels, to your gut and immune system. These pathways can all be mapped scientifically. The challenge is to open up and travel these pathways in your mind and your body through self-knowledge.

Get to know what sets off your different emotional states and then learn to deal with them effectively. What triggers your anger, what gives you joy, what creates a great deal of mental strain for you?

To get to this level of self-awareness or emotional self-knowledge may require the help of a professional. A few sessions with a counsellor or a psychologist will highlight why you feel and respond the way you do. Learning some form of meditation or technique that allows you to be still and go inward is another effective method to gain insight and awareness.

By focusing on self-knowledge, you will become conscious of your mood changes, your thought patterns, your negative beliefs. Try to begin to identify the triggers.

Possible emotional triggers

Something as simple as your **menstrual cycle** may be a major trigger. Once you begin to identify your recurrent weepiness, anxiety or irritability as always occurring prior to your period and then passing, it becomes easy to let it go. Then you can allow yourself some extra rest and pampering and avoid certain things for that period of time. The emotional symptoms themselves become less important. You have an understanding that they are triggered by hormonal changes beyond your control and you can implement a few strategies to ease your state of mind.

Sleep deprivation is another powerful trigger for a mood slump. A heavy work schedule, a sick child, a deadline and a few nights without sleep is a sure way to set off an emotional roller coaster of anger, hostility and even a depressed mood. The explanation for this is that your brain's output of neurotransmitters may become depleted with sleep deprivation, leaving you feeling miserable.

Hypoglycaemia (a drop in blood sugar) from skipping meals or going beyond three to four hours without a snack is a powerful trigger for emotional turbulence. You may not even know that things as simple as skipping meals may spark off your feelings of anger. An excessive amount of alcohol or even one tot more than you are used to may generate physical fatigue, excessive moodiness and negative thought patterns.

The company of **certain people** may even elicit your mood changes or energy slumps. By being aware of this, you can simply move away from them. If this is not possible, consciously take charge of your perceptions and do not allow them to disturb your equilibrium.

Some people are more sensitive to certain triggers than others. What are you most sensitive to? Be proactive about trying to prevent these situations occurring. If this is not possible, you can at least cushion the blow with a few tools. A session at the gym after work or a 20-minute catnap on your desk or a energising freshly squeezed juice may just help out and even shift your mood before you plunge into a downward spiral.

However, there are certainly life situations which you cannot alter. Suffering from or caring for someone with a terminal illness, being stuck in an unhappy marriage, dealing with a disabled child or living with your own depression are circumstances beyond your control. Nevertheless, it is still worthwhile identifying the factors that worsen the accompanying emotional and mental states.

Many emotions are also deeply rooted. You may carry anger and resentment within you due to life traumas or have various reasons for a low self-esteem. With these deeper emotions, it is even more important to identify and begin to understand them truly and their triggers so that healing can begin to take place.

Letting go

True empowerment is an unusual combination of humility and surrender, together with self-confidence and personal responsibility. It seems as though these two concepts –'taking charge' and 'letting go' – are mutually exclusive. But it is exactly the blend of these two that will bring about empowered living for you. Have the confidence to steer your own path while possessing the humility to trust God and surrender to the universe.

Taking charge of your life and your health does not mean you now enter the downward spiral of self-blame and guilt when things do not work out. As much as you need to take personal responsibility for everything within your grasp, there is a spiritual component beyond you. The world beyond your control demands some degree of surrender as you may have learnt from Jeanne's personal healing story.

It is very difficult explaining how to let go. It demands a confidence and internal strength to surrender to 'the bigger picture'. Most importantly, it requires a conscious 'head' decision.

There are so many things you may need to let go of: your control over others, your need for perfection, your need for approval, relationships that no longer serve you, the need to know and understand it all, but most importantly your anger, bitterness, resentment and need for revenge.

Persistent unforgiveness is part of human nature, but not being able to let go and forgive appears to work to the detriment not only of your spiritual wellbeing but also your physical health. The state of unforgiveness (or *not letting go*) is a powerful mixture of bitterness, anger, hostility, resentment and fear. These have a powerful negative effect on your heart, neurological function and immunity.

Dr Dean Ornish, the US cardiologist and lifestyle guru, explains:'When I talk about forgiveness, I mean *letting go*, not excusing the other person or condoning their behaviour. Just letting go of your own suffering.'

Authenticity

To take charge you also need to live a life of truth. Being authentic is perhaps one of the key ingredients in your physical and spiritual health. The qualities of honesty and integrity are the cornerstones of personal power.

You have an inner world and an outer world. When these two are not matched, there is a serious imbalance. When there is a disconnection between what you are truly feeling and thinking and what you are portraying to the world, a betrayal takes place. Not only are you betraying your true self but you are also betraying your body. Your body picks up this imbalance and manifests stress, fatigue, exhaustion and compromise to your immunity. Your personal power is simply draining out of your system and making you exhausted. You cannot fool your body. You obviously have a sacred part of your inner world that is not to be shared with all. However, what you do share of yourself with your outside world needs to be your authentic self.

You can literally get ill from living an inauthentic life. You may spend your life trying to please and satisfy others. Approval does indeed feel good. The problem is that in your pursuit of approval, so much of your inner world needs to be buried. You build your life on what you think others are expecting of you and thereby expend too much energy in maintaining this. The reality is that your perceptions of what you think they think or want from you are often false and you slowly but surely lose contact with your essence and your inner truth.

To truly access personal power requires you to live an authentic life, one in which your inner and outer worlds are congruent.

Take charge of your physical health

Preventive health care is the method whereby you put the concepts of 'empower' and 'take charge' into practice. This is where the philosophy is translated into action.

Thirty years ago, doctors were certainly not focused on preventive care. Now in the 21st century, science and medicine have a clear understanding of the causes of many chronic diseases. Several of these illnesses are called 'chronic diseases of lifestyle' because it is indeed lifestyle factors which can cause disease and ill health. Although your doctor has a duty to advise and direct you in the implementation of preventive care, your health is essentially your responsibility. This is where you can best practice taking charge of your life! You live at a time in the history of modern medicine when your implementation of effective health measures can make a significant difference. *You* have the capacity to lead a life that is compatible with good health.

Although this sounds like common sense, most women remain in the dark. The reasons for this may include information overload, confusion,

Table 1: Levels of prevention

	Prevention	What to do	Examples
Level 1 Primary prevention	Healthy lifestyle factors	Smart ways to live well	Stop smoking Exercise Optimal nutrition Moderate alcohol Manage obesity
Level 2 Primary prevention	Early detection of illness	Screening	Pap smears Breast self-exam Mammograms Blood pressure Glucose HIV test
Level 3 Secondary prevention	Early management of problems/risk factors	Treat problems and risk factors: medically and with lifestyle changes	Treat high blood pressure with: ☆ medication if required ☆ moderate exercise ☆ diet modification
Level 4 Tertiary prevention	Early and active management of disease	Prevent further development of disease by implementing lifestyle changes and ensuring good medical care	Diabetes, HIV/AIDS, heart disease, early cancer

poor access to accurate information or time constraints during consultations with doctors. Ideally, you would like to ensure that you never get ill. Unfortunately this is not always possible but there is much that is within your control. Prevention is so much more than the deterrence of all illnesses. It consists of many tiers of care and intervention.

Your personal Health Action Plan

Six-month plan

Month 1: Take charge EMPOWER
Week 1: Journal and family history
Week 2: Life stages: screening
Week 3: Health parameters
Week 4: Lifestyle habits

Month 2: Take care EMBRACE
Week 1: Get out of your head and into your heart! (CARDIAC check)
Week 2: Nurturing the nurturer!
Week 3: Take good care
Week 4: Nurture your beauty, nurture your sexuality

Month 3: Take action EAT The SELF diet
Week 1: Empower and embrace – eating
Week 2: Eat and exercise – essentials
Week 3: Energy in your food
Week 4: Enrich your diet

Month 4: Take action EXERCISE
Week 1: The start
Week 2: Build up
Week 3: Sustain
Week 4: Keep moving

Month 5: Take action ENERGISE (Stress management)
Week 1: Rest and sleep
Week 2: Breath
Week 3: Meditation and other stuff
Week 4: Pace your life

Month 6: Take action ENRICH
Week 1: Meditate
Week 2: Write your own personal prescription
Week 3: Spiritual nutrients
Week 4: Action

Practical plan ✿

JUST AS YOU would create a business plan or school lift scheme, the task ahead is to create your own health and life strategy. Since you are now in the driver's seat, you need a map and directions. I call this 'map' a 'HAP': a **Health Action Plan.**

With more people becoming interested in their health, you may find in books, in publications, in your local gym or through your medical scheme many different programmes or wellness strategies. Unfortunately these programmes are usually 'one size fits all' for women and another perhaps for men or children. Can you imagine a *one size fits all* bra for all women?

You are an individual woman with a family history, a medical profile, a set of physical parameters, a lifestyle and emotional make-up that is unique. Your health plan needs to be tailored to your age, life stage and individuality. You may therefore take this Health Action Plan and make it your own **personal** Health Action Plan.

This plan is about the rest of your life, so there is no quick fix.

This plan is a six-month programme. Each chapter of this book has a one-month programme around the subject of that chapter. You can choose to implement it as you wish. It is going to be your personal plan. It is, however, best to start with Chapter 1, choosing to structure it to suit your needs. You can either do it month-by-month, week-by-week, following the topics in the book according to chapter and month. Alternatively, you may wish to implement more than one aspect at a time. For example, you may want to begin the programme for eating and exercising and energising all at the same time within the same month. Feel free to do that! All you do is combine the activity for Week 1 of eating, Week 1 of exercising and Week 1 of energy, and so on.

⚹
Month 1:
Take charge

Week 1:
Journal, family
history and risk
factors

1.1 The SELF
journal
⚹

Get started

✦ You need a recording system for your Personal Health Action Plan.

✦ You can choose to do this on paper or electronically.

✦ Purchase for your Health Action Plan a colourful or an inspirational journal or open up a folder on your computer entitled 'My Personal Health Action Plan'. Call it the SELF journal.

✦ Start today: Make a note on today's date *'Made decision today to take charge of my health and life'* .

✦ Create goals for yourself. Write down in your journal five short-term and five long-term goals. Writing is a powerful method to transform the intangible into concrete results.

Create a Take Charge chart

Make a head decision each day to implement one idea. Thoughts are real things.

The intention to internalise an idea and the acquisition of knowledge creates an internal power.

Table 2

a. Take charge of WHAT?

	To do
My life	Make a head decision 'I am the driver'
My perceptions	★ Open up to a new world view of courage and trust in yourself ★ Examine your core beliefs ★ Choose positive, realistic, affirming actions
My time	★ Create 'white space' in your calendar ★ Stop complaining – create 'your time' ★ Create gaps before and after each task. Sandwich each activity between five minutes of 'nothing' on either side

Table 2 (continued)
a. Take charge of WHAT?

	To do
My relationships	★ Stop self-blame ★ Choose good company ★ Become a better listener ★ Keep your word ★ Be self-reliant ★ Show appreciation
My body	★ Understand how it works ★ Appreciate how it works ★ Say 'yes' or 'no' to decisions involving your body
My personal health	★ Know your family history ★ Know your risk factors ★ Know your health parameters ★ Know the screening/disease detection required for your life stage ★ Implement lifestyle change

Table 3
a. Take charge HOW?

Understand your body Understand healing	Read Search Internet Ask questions Develop relationship with doctor
Understand emotional/ mental health	Become conscious of your mood changes Seek professional help Identify your common triggers ★ Menstrual cycle ★ Sleep deprivation ★ Hunger and hypoglycaemia ★ Reactions to different people
Let go	Practice forgiveness Let go of guilt and anger Meditate
Be authentic	Choose honesty and integrity Allow yourself imperfections

᠕
1.2 Family history

Get to know
these facts
᠕

+ Your family doctor will at some stage have asked many questions about your family medical history. But it is very important for **you** to know and understand these facts, too.

+ It is important to identify the family illnesses, so that you can detect them early and make the necessary lifestyle adjustments.

+ There is a metaphor that describes the relationship between genetic and environmental factors in the development of disease. The loaded gun is your genetics and family history. Pulling the trigger is your lifestyle choices. You may have a genetic predisposition to heart disease. If you choose to smoke, become overweight and live a sedentary lifestyle there is a strong likelihood that you will 'pull the trigger' and develop a heart attack. If you take charge, implement exercise, good nutrition and weight management, and stop smoking, you may alter your destiny!

᠕
Do you have
a family history
of?
᠕

+ Heart disease, angina, stroke, or vascular disease
+ Hypertension (high blood pressure)
+ High cholesterol
+ Diabetes
+ Breast cancer
+ Colon cancer

Having a positive family history of disease does not mean that you will get that sickness. It is merely a guide to encourage you to be proactive particularly in that area. Family history is only one risk factor among many.

᠕
1.3 Risk factors

Get to know
your other risk
factors
᠕

Are you at risk for?

HEART DISEASE

Major risk factors
+ hypertension
+ diabetes
+ high cholesterol

- ✦ smoking
- ✦ family history
- ✦ obesity

Minor risk factors

- ✦ stress
- ✦ inactivity
- ✦ huge abdominal girth

BREAST CANCER

- ✦ family history
- ✦ no pregnancies or lactation
- ✦ advanced age pregnancies

OSTEOPOROSIS

- ✦ smoking
- ✦ inactivity (lack of exercise)
- ✦ small frame (underweight)
- ✦ caucasian (light skinned)
- ✦ poor diet – insufficient calcium

Please remember: Risk factors DO NOT mean you will get the illness. They are a guide for you to become proactive.

✕
Week 2:
Your life stages

Screening

✕

Check out the relevant tables below according to your particular age and make a list of what screening tests you may need to have. Make the appointments this week even if you schedule them for the near future. Make sure they take place within this six-month plan!

20-40s

You are busy rearing a family and/or building a career now and it can be stressful but this is when you should be at your peak health; you are young, fit and strong. During this time, common problems include hormonal disturbances, stress-related diseases, fertility, pregnancy, childbirth and sexual problems, STDs, depression, and perhaps chronic illnesses may begin. Many women also gain weight during the childbirth years, which they have difficulty shaking off.

Table 4

20-40 Health screening

Investigation	Frequency
Breast self-examination	Monthly
Clinical breast exam (doctor)	Annually
Pap smear	Every one to two years
Blood pressure	Every two years
Cholesterol	Baseline (possibly every five years)
Glucose	Baseline (possibly every five years)
HIV testing	Baseline (and thereafter discuss with doctor)
Physical examination	Every four to five years
Skin self-examination	Monthly

40-60s

This is when the lifestyle you have chosen will become most apparent in your state of health. Now is the time that the effects of bad habits show: smoking 40 cigarettes a day is likely to result in wrinkles and lung problems, a lack of exercise can translate into weight problems and/or Type 2 diabetes.

But it is never too late to implement a healthy lifestyle. Even once you have reached the age group of 40-60, your body can still reap the benefits of a healthy living plan. It is also a time of making peace with yourself and pursuing your own interests.

Common problems women encounter at this age include heart problems, blood pressure changes, weight gain, osteoporosis, menopause, loss of libido and stress.

Table 5

40-60 Health screening

Investigation	Frequency
Breast self-examination	Monthly
Clinical breast exam (doctor)	Annually
Pap smear	Every one to two years
Blood pressure	Every two years
Cholesterol	Baseline (possibly every five years)
Glucose	Baseline (possibly every five years)
HIV testing	Baseline (and thereafter discuss with doctor)
Physical examination	Every four to five years
Mammogram	Annually
Bone density testing	Baseline from 50 (earlier if indicated); annually if problem detected
Fecal blood	Annually
Skin self-examination	Monthly

60+

If you have always been healthy, there is no reason why this stage in your life should be any different. However, there are certain things which you should look out for.

Conditions associated with ageing include arthritis, heart disease, cancer, stroke, osteoporosis and rheumatoid arthritis, and many women are prone to depression during this time in their life. But the good news is that your choice of lifestyle plays a big part in how healthy you are in this stage of your life.

Medical science has also advanced enormously, and treatment for several diseases, that would not have been an option even a decade ago, is now possible. Important things

Table 6

60+ Health screening

Investigation	Frequency
Breast self-examination	Monthly
Clinical breast exam (doctor)	Annually
Pap smear	Annually
Blood pressure	Annually
Cholesterol	Possibly every two to five years; if abnormal, at least yearly
Glucose	Possibly yearly
Physical examination	Annually
Mammogram	Annually
Fecal blood	Annually
Urine analysis	Annually
Skin self-examination	Monthly
Eye examination	Annually
Hearing test	Annually

you can do during this time of your life to prevent many of these diseases include improving your circulation with regular, moderate exercise and eating a low-fat diet that contains lots of fruit and vegetables. The important thing is to stay active, both mentally and physically, as this definitely slows down the ageing process.

✿

Week 3: Document your physical parameters ✿

This week make a list of what parameters you need to get checked. (You may not have access to this information until your visit to your doctor or when the tests are done. So you do not have to get them urgently. You simply need to draw up the list.)

Get to know these parameters in the next few months and perhaps record some of them in your SELF journal, together with dates of screening and test results.

1. Blood pressure
2. Cholesterol
3. Glucose
4. Weight
5. Body Mass Index (see Chapter 4) or body fat percentage
6. Blood group (in case of accident or need for blood transfusion)
7. HIV status. It is so much more comfortable to stay in denial, but the sooner you know your status the better. If you are HIV-positive, the sooner you are able to begin therapy, the better your chances of living a long and good life on medication.

Week 4: Your lifestyle HABITS

This week draw up a list of all your unhealthy lifestyle habits. Choose to address one bad habit per month for these next six months.

When starting a health plan, most people tend to strengthen the areas which are already good and neglect the bad habits. For example, if you are quite focused on exercise, you will run off to the gym this week and add extra time to your programme. That is not what you should do now. Choose to really focus on the weaker areas.

Examples of bad habits:

1. Smoking – Think of all the damage you are doing to your body. Consider attending a smoking cessation programme or using a nicotine substitute in the form of skin patch or gum to wean you off the addiction. Discuss with your doctor.
2. Alcohol – Drinking in moderation may be good for you and your heart. One glass of red wine a day is beneficial. Beyond two tots a day is extremely harmful

to your liver, your brain and beyond. Choose to cut
down to not more than one tot per day.

3. Excessive stimulants – Too much caffeine as found in
coffee, cola drinks and chocolate upsets your body
balance. Try to replace some cups of coffee with herbal
teas. Drink more water instead of fizzy colas.

4. Convenience foods – Many processed food contains
harmful fats, refined flour and sugar as well as
artificial additives and preservatives, which can
provoke biochemical chaos and deplete your energy
(see Chapter 4). Cut back on take-outs.

5. Crash dieting – This is a poor lifestyle habit! Choose to
let go of this continuous crash dieting approach and
get onto the Chapter 3 programme. Fad diets are
poorly balanced and deplete the body of vital
nutrients.

CHAPTER 2

Embrace

Introduction

A pair of lovers holding each other so close that they can feel the other's heartbeat. An infant wrapped securely within the arms of his mother, head resting against her breasts.

These are the images conjured up when you think of an embrace.

An embrace is a circle, a contained place of love. Close to your heart, close to your breast. Try and replace the image of the lovers or the infant and imagine yourself in the centre of this space. It is a space in which you are held and loved. You are secure, recognised, accepted and understood.

Isn't this what we all yearn for? Don't you wish there was someone out there who could do this all for you? This chapter will encourage you to shift those expectations from others and rather begin to nurture yourself. Although you may have a loving partner and warm friends, only you can really do it. And when you do begin to embrace yourself, you will trigger a cascade of events that manifests in a great deal of personal health and satisfaction.

The theme of the previous chapter – to *empower* and take charge of your health – entails a rational 'head' decision. To now *embrace* yourself requires of you to move into your heart. The heart dimension is a metaphor for compassion and caring. The heart is literally the centre of your life force and is described as the seat of your emotions. This chapter provides an extensive review of your emotions, their connection to your body and the fundamental role they play in your health. It encourages you to truly take care of yourself. To embrace yourself requires a process of accepting all your faults and imperfections. This allows you to begin to nurture yourself, celebrate your life, make peace with your body, feel and experience your emotions, and indulge your interests and passions.

Healing professionals and even medically trained people have for the most part accepted that emotions are essential components of wellbeing and healing. How nurturing and embracing yourself enhances your health and your body's healing capacity has become much clearer in the past few years. Surprisingly, when you truly embrace yourself, you open up the channels that allow others to begin to nurture and embrace you, too.

Grace's story

It is 6 a.m. on the 1st of January: my first day as a fully fledged doctor. My first real patient! In Medical Ward 6 the care of patients is being handed over from the intern of 1987 to the intern of 1988: me!

The intern of '87 tells me (in front of my new patient) that Grace is a very difficult patient. She has been admitted to this ward three times in the past two weeks, each time for a suspected heart attack. Each time the electrocardiogram (ECG) reveals a serious arrhythmia (unstable abnormal heart rhythm) and possibly unstable angina. Grace is only 43 and is the mother of young children. She is slim and attractive but seems agitated. She does have high blood pressure but has no other major risk factors and has no previous heart disease.

Intern '87 tells me why Grace is so difficult. *'She demands an explanation for everything. She wants to know what every test means and whether it has to be done. She will not allow any procedure to be performed without her permission. She is driving us and the nursing staff crazy'.*

'Isn't it her right to know these things?' I ask.

'She shouldn't be so pushy! Who is the doctor here? Can't she just leave us alone without all this discussion and let me get on with my work? We just cannot seem to reverse this arrhythmia. She is also so forceful and assertive,' he complains.

I have to be at the hospital for at least another 10 hours today with few clinical skills and even less confidence. I sit down uncomfortably on the stool next to Grace's bed and begin to take a full medical history. She is indeed a strong woman and as she speaks she exudes a real toughness.

She explains all her symptoms and the unfolding of her medical situation with clarity and exceptional detail. She tells me about her demanding management role in a mining company as well as her responsibility as a mother of young children. (So far I can relate, having left my twelve-week-old infant in the care of someone as I embark on my year's internship.) She seems completely in control and stoical.

On New Year's day in 1988 at 6.30 a.m., I am not going anywhere beyond the confines of this hospital and since I have only one patient, I continue to sit next to Grace and try rather naïvely to make conversation. This goes on for about 15 minutes (which feels like 15 hours) until I enquire whether she is married or has a love in her life. Suddenly the floodgates burst open. She sobs and weeps uncontrollably for a long while before she begins talking. My instinct is to jump up and run away! No manual or tutorial in seven years of training provided a protocol for what to do now.

She tells me how her husband died tragically in a car accident eight months previously. She tries to express the magnitude of her pain and her grief. She describes how she cannot cope with this weakness, this vulnerability, this heartache and so as of a few weeks ago she decided to 'buck up'. Grace explains that being 'tough' and strong has always worked for her in all areas of her life. She describes how, as she became numb, she literally felt herself turning to stone.

Shortly thereafter these frightening chest pains and palpitations began and this recurring arrhythmia now seems resistant to the cardiologist's treatment. Each time the condition settled, she would be discharged and a few days later returned as an emergency. With this hospital admission nothing was reversing the pain, the disturbed rhythm or the abnormal findings on the ECG. The cardiac staff were now considering inserting a pacemaker and were awaiting further clinical discussions.

Grace continued to sob as she described the love that she shared with her childhood sweetheart over a period of 25 years and all her dreams she had still hoped would come true. She cried for a long time, interspersed with some laughs about the past, and then we sat in silence for another long while.

The following day on the grand round, the clinical chief explained to the entourage of physicians, registrars, nurses and to us the juniors that he was baffled. Grace's arrhythmia (and chest pains) had disappeared without any change in medication. He was discharging her but was sure she would be wheeled into the hospital again in a few days. Grace returned to the outpatient clinic after two weeks free of chest pains. The abnormal heart rhythms never returned. She continued her hospital visits monthly and then six-monthly without any sign of abnormality. I remained at that hospital for three years after my internship so I continued to see Grace intermittently.

The fact that Grace's arrhythmia reversed or settled or disappeared is not a phenomenon from the realm of the miraculous and supernatural. It may not happen as often as we would like, but people do heal unexpectedly from all kinds of conditions and one of the areas that affects this healing is dealing with and releasing emotional blockages.

Grace initiated my real medical education when she told me that 'she had melted her heart of stone' and was allowing herself to be vulnerable at the same time as being powerful. She was trying to take real care of herself and her emotions too. It would be at least a decade before I would begin to read in medical journals about the therapeutic value of patients being assertive and questioning, that emotions profoundly affect the physical body and that as a doctor you can help heal illness if you just sit and listen.

Note: At about the same time that I was a medical student and performing my internship, journal articles were being written describing the relationship between emotions and illness, as well as patients just like Grace, in New Haven Connecticut by a surgeon with revolutionary thinking. Dr Bernie Siegel called these people (approximately ten per cent of his patients) ECPs: exceptional patients. He describes an ECP as:

✦ insisting on being treated with dignity
✦ being assertive with doctors, demanding information, wanting to participate in decision making
✦ questions and prods for more knowledge

♦ possibly defiant – these patients have a much greater chance of survival and healing from illness than submissive, accepting patients.

My story

Growing up, I always had a sense of some power and meaning in my internal feelings. But at school, power and meaning were measured in achievement of the best results and being pretty and popular. Although my results were more than okay, being in a class with super-bright kids and friendly with gorgeous girls made me feel rather mediocre. My internal feelings were never identified or explained. I often felt as invisible as this internal sensation.

Years later, through training at medical school, things seemed worse. Structure, function and pure science ruled my world for many years. The world that dictates measurement and research did not allow for internal feelings of power or meaning. *'Detach, don't feel too much, don't get emotional with patients'* was the unspoken rule. The dominant message of this world view in which I was being schooled was that the biology of the body (or disease) is overwhelmingly important and that thoughts, feelings and emotions are insignificant events. (I now know that these feelings and emotions are the very fundamentals of which all life is composed.)

In the middle of a tutorial involving a child with cancer, I would run to the bathroom to hide my tears and then return secretly to hug the child. I was a closet 'touchy-feely' – not the best type to get ahead as a medical student. I would faint at the sight of a septic amputation and awake to the tug of my professor and his patronising words: *'Medical training is not for the faint-hearted, lovey!'*

So often, I witnessed that my patient's clinical outcome did not follow the textbook case. Some patients would not get better, despite the best medical treatment and others, given no hope, would recover. I felt that there was always something deeper within the healing or the illness of my patients, just as there was within me.

The many years of rearing five children, interspersed with the taking care of patients, have been filled with pain, joy, personal triumphs as well as personal failures. My profound teachers (my patients and my children) have guided me to embrace and understand that this internal power, this mixture of emotions and thoughts and senses, is more complex than human anatomy and cannot be dissected in the same way. This power is as much about vulnerability and softness as it is about potency and strength. You, too, have an immeasurable force within you, perhaps residing within the core of your embrace – within your heart. And by embracing it and nurturing it, you will begin to live with greater health and meaning.

Take heart

To embrace yourself and take special care of your health requires a journey to the centre of your body – to your heart. You need to get out of your head and into your heart. Like me, you may be baffled by this notion. My approach is always to retreat into my head, into a formal space that thinks instead of feels. It is a safe retreat. You may do the same. But the mind is ultimately a less gratifying place than the heart. Your heart is the place of nurturing and healing.

What is your heart?

Your heart is a muscle pump, literally the powerhouse of your body. It is located behind your breastbone, mainly on the left side of your chest. It consists of three layers – a pericardium on the outside, an endocardium on the inside and a thick muscle layer called the myocardium in the middle, and is divided into four chambers called the two atria and the two ventricles.

The heart functions in a cycle of contraction and relaxation. During contraction, blood is pumped out of your heart. Then the heart muscle relaxes before the next heartbeat. This allows blood to fill your heart again. Every organ in your body depends on your heart to pump and supply the essential oxygen-rich blood.

Have you ever wondered what makes your heart beat? An electrical system in your heart has the ability to generate electrical activity on its own. This produces electrical waves that can be measured in the form of an electrocardiogram (ECG). This gives doctors information about your heart's function. The heart, just like any other organ, requires blood to supply it with oxygen and other nutrients so that it can do its work as a muscle pump. It gets its blood from coronary arteries that carry blood to the heart muscle.

Heart disease is the number one killer of both men and women in most parts of the world. You may make the mistake of thinking of heart disease as a male concern, but ten times more women die from heart attacks than from breast cancer per year. Female hormones do protect women from heart disease but only until menopause, when the risk increases sharply.

However, coronary disease does not just suddenly happen when you reach 50. Your negative lifestyle habits, such as smoking, obesity, inactivity and bad nutrition, as well as your mindset and emotions, help lay down the fatty plaques indicative of artery disease.

Angina reveals that coronary vessels are partially blocked and too little oxygen is reaching the heart, manifesting as a crushing pain. This is worsened by exercise and emotional turmoil. A myocardial infarct, commonly called a 'heart attack' or 'coronary', means that one or more of the vessels had become blocked enough to cut off the blood and oxygen supply to the heart muscle. A portion of the heart muscle 'dies' in the process. Internalised stress, too, can exacerbate heart disease and precipitate heart attacks.

Emotional and spiritual heart

Your heart is a muscle pump that certainly needs to be addressed physically – but you also have an emotional and a spiritual heart dimension. Your heart is a metaphor for the seat of your emotions and the seat of your soul. The association of heart with emotions is, however, more than a metaphor, as there is a scientific explanation for this.

The reason why your physical heart responds so strongly to emotional turmoil is because it is so closely connected to the autonomic nervous system. This is the nervous system that controls all body and organ functions, including your heart, lungs, your digestive tract, your hormones and believe it or not, sexual arousal too. This nervous system is divided into a sympathetic branch and a parasympathetic branch.

You should know for certain that emotions affect your heart – suffer a fright and your heart pounds. Get angry and your blood pressure rises. But it is not just anger and anxiety. Science is also showing that desperation and depression also have a huge effect. When you begin to feel an emotion such as anger or fear, there is a stimulus to your sympathetic nervous system eliciting an outpouring of chemicals which actually causes the vessels to tighten. Joy and love stimulate the other part of this nervous system (parasympathetic) and this causes an opening of the blood vessels, allowing more blood to flow to your heart muscle.

This does not mean that you should never feel or express fear or anger. These feelings need to be felt and expressed for the good of your health. Damage occurs when a negative emotion, such as anger, is constantly present. This maintains the sympathetic nervous systems on full charge and the adrenalin and other hormones continue flowing relentlessly. You need to feel the emotions, deal with them, express them healthily and then let them go. When the emotional heart and spiritual heart begin to open, then the physical heart often follows. In this sense, blocked hearts and heart attacks may mirror your emotional life and the ability to manage your feelings.

The heart as language

The relationship between your heart and your emotions is integrated into your everyday language. You often use the word 'heart' in describing yourselves and others. You experience 'heartache' and 'heart-throbs'. You describe loving individuals as being 'big-hearted' or 'warm-hearted'. If someone is cold, you may say she has 'no heart' or that a brave and courageous person has a 'lot of heart'. Interestingly, the word for heart in French is *couer*, the root of the word 'courage'. When you express all your emotions and let it all out 'You are wearing your heart on your sleeve.' It all seems like warm fuzzy stuff, whereas in fact these metaphors are translated into your body pathways. When life is so painful and you need to shut off emotion, you may tell yourself to 'harden your heart'. This is exactly what may happen at a physical level when you suppress what you really feel, as I witnessed 17 years ago with my very first patient, Grace.

Emotional health

You generally feel one of the four main basic emotions at any time: *anger, sadness, fear or happiness.* The two others are classified as *love and shame.* All other emotions are shades of these basic emotions. For example, rage is part of anger whereas anxiety and panic are manifestations of fear. Despair, grief and depression are classifications of sadness.

You may think of an emotion as ephemeral or invisible just because you cannot measure it in the same way as you can take your pulse. But emotions are really part of your survival equipment. They're an essential part of the mechanism by which you regulate your life. Negative emotions are not always pathological and may play a positive role in your wellbeing. For example, anxiety is a drive that helps you to avoid real or invisible threats and you would never meet deadlines without it. Fear keeps you away from real danger, but is destructive when it becomes unrelenting due to only perceived danger. The challenge is to let the anxiety or fear go once the deadline or the threat is over.

The word 'emotion' contains within it the word 'motion', to move (from the Latin, meaning to move forward). If you do not do the moving forward, the emotions may do the moving for you. They may accelerate and cause cells within the body to move in a certain direction or take on a pattern of illness.

You may not even recognise your feelings. You may walk around feeling sad without even knowing that you are sad or why you feel the way you do. Our society often encourages a detachment from certain feelings. What happens is that the 'motion' – the energy inherent in a feeling – needs to go somewhere. It can become a physical symptom, such as abdominal pain or a headache, which are much easier to complain about than feeling sad.

Worse is when sadness becomes transformed into a more 'acceptable' emotion such as anger. Anger can be an ugly emotion but an angry person is often accepted as driven, aggressive, demanding or even a 'go-getter'. These attributes are sometimes valued in the workplace. This is more common in men but found in women to some degree too. It is often just deep sadness that goes unidentified or has not been confronted for long periods that become transformed into fury or resentment. If you carry any of these damaging emotions or have unresolved sorrow, you need to be concerned about the physical effect on your heart and to your whole body.

Anger, aggression, loneliness, passion or love may be at the root of what makes you sick and what makes you well. Studies reveal that following retirement, the incidence of heart attacks quadruples and following the loss of a loved one, it rises significantly. A study on hopelessness and helplessness found that people who think of themselves as failures have far more heart attacks than their optimistic counterparts.

Where are emotions located in the body?

That emotions affect your health is hardly news. But this relationship between emotions and your physical body is turning out to be far more interesting than you could have imagined! Emotions actually have their source in the physical brain. However, new research is revealing how alike and in what close proximity the emotional control centres are to purely physical control centres. So the part of your brain controlling the feeling of love may be the very same or similar to that controlling your digestive tract.

Scientists using sophisticated brain imaging technology are learning what goes on inside the brain when you experience emotion – a subject once dismissed as too abstract for serious research.

In the latest investigation, neurologists at the University of Iowa College of Medicine, have shown how feelings of anger, sadness, happiness and fear are linked to distinct patterns in specific regions of the brain. This study offers some laboratory evidence to back up the fact that emotions, and ultimately consciousness itself, are intimately linked to vital body systems.

It seems that most emotions can be traced to the very same brain regions that control regulation and balance of things as physical as blood pressure, body temperature and hormonal activity. The big difference now is that neurologists have the tools to see what a 'feeling brain' looks like.

Through scans called PET (Positron Emission Tomography), brain regions activated or deactivated during each of four 'primary' emotional states – anger, sadness, happiness and fear – can be mapped. You are not sensing emotion with some bizarre brain structures. You are feeling with the same structures used to regulate the balance of your whole life.

Emotional distress can cause physical pain

We all know that physical pain causes you emotional distress. For example, living with a chronically painful back may cause you to feel depressed. Or just think of those labour pains and the emotional turmoil they cause! It is clear that pain triggers an emotional response.

Remarkably, this 'new science' demonstrates that the reverse is also true: emotional distress can be physically painful. Depressed people are three times more likely to suffer from chronic pain, according to recent research. If you are struggling with either depression or pain, there is a good chance you have both. This link between sensory pain and emotional pain is rooted in the nervous system. Both are governed by the same neurotransmitters (nerve proteins) such as serotonin, adrenalin and substance P, and both are processed in the same part of the brain.

When the whole circuit is working properly, pain and emotional anguish are self-limiting, i.e. they will stop. The feelings fade and life goes on. But if the circuit is malfunctioning or if a problem persists for a long time, the brain's distress signals stay switched on. One study found that a person with recurrent migraines was five times more likely to suffer from depression than non-migraine sufferers.

The good news is that treating chronic pain can often alleviate depression and the same is true for treating depression. The pain often subsides. It is always useful to use mind-body techniques as well as medical therapy. Modalities such as meditation, hypnosis and imagery may help interrupt this interminable circuit of emotional and physical pain.

Whole-body illnesses

A host of illnesses cannot be treated by curing the body or the mind or the emotions individually. I call these whole-body illnesses because they involve your body, mood and thoughts all at the same time. You cannot just view one dimension of these conditions in the way you could treat a broken toe. Ideally, all illnesses or imbalances should be seen as whole-body disorders, but with the following maladies the imbalance in emotions, in thoughts and in physical symptoms are all overtly apparent together. (For a full clinical review of each section, see Chapter 7.)

Depression
Clinical depression can affect your physical wellbeing, commonly resulting in sleep problems, chronic fatigue and loss of appetite, as well as persistent headaches, digestive disorders or chronic pain. It affects your mood, with feelings of sadness, emptiness, hopelessness, irritability and especially a loss of libido. It affects the way you think and interferes with your concentration and decision making.

Anxiety
An anxiety disorder seriously disturbs your sleep, it can make you irritable and undermine your ability to concentrate and think clearly. This constant fearful feeling keeps your adrenaline pumping, your heart racing and your palms sweating. People with generalised anxiety disorder have physical symptoms that are so pronounced that they frequently first seek treatment with a medical doctor or specialist – most often a cardiologist as they complain of palpitations and chest pain.

Eating disorders (Anorexia and Bulimia)
Real eating disorders are amongst the most deadly of all mental illnesses and among the most difficult to treat. They involve serious disturbances in eating behaviour, such as extreme and unhealthy reduction of food intake or severe overeating, as well as emotional distress such as depression and anxiety. The sufferer has seriously disturbed thought patterns completely out of sync with reality. Physical body function is often affected – most commonly with kidney, liver and thyroid problems, and even heart disorders in the most extreme cases.

Chronic Fatigue Syndrome (CFS)
CFS is a syndrome that describes varying combinations of symptoms including recurrent fatigue, sore throats, low-grade fever, muscle and

joint pain, headaches, loss of concentration and often features of depression. Although still somewhat controversial within the medical profession, CFS is not a new disease at all. CFS is often not taken seriously enough by many doctors who may not believe that it is a real condition at all (see Chapter 5).

There is absolutely no shame in developing any of these conditions. You did not bring this upon yourself. In the same way as anaemia or high blood pressure needs proper medical attention, so does depression, an anxiety or eating disorder or CFS.

Emotional centres throughout you body – Chakras

From a scientific viewpoint, you can now understand how emotions originate in brain matter and are intricately connected to your physical body. Against this Western scientific backdrop, it is interesting to consider an Eastern view of emotions that has crept into our world view.

You may have heard of the term 'chakras'. Either you know all about chakras and have embraced this way of thinking or you may dismiss it as a New Age development and not your scene.

So what are chakras all about? This fascinating Indian philosophy spanning a few thousand years simply explains where emotions are located in your physical body and how they affect your emotional and physical health.

Seven emotional centres, each connected to an anatomical structure in your body, are described. Each centre encompasses a particular group of organs and is associated with a set of emotions. Each is thought to control energy flow around the body, and contains the contrasting aspects of that particular set of emotions. What this means is that the emotion is expressed either in terms of *power* or *vulnerability*. The power side of the emotion is what makes you more powerful and strong in the outer world. The vulnerability aspect actually endows you with a power and strength in your inner world.

Note: This thinking actually matches the sentiment of Chapter 1. To empower yourself and take charge is to balance that power or strength in your outer world with that of your vulnerability (being authentic, letting go, etc) in your inner world.

In each centre, you can determine whether most of your strength and health is connected to the power side or to the vulnerability side. For optimum health you need a balance of both. If you have an imbalance between the two or only one side of the emotion, then this philosophy plus scientific research suggests that you are setting the scene for susceptibility to illness in the organs connected to that emotional centre. (The

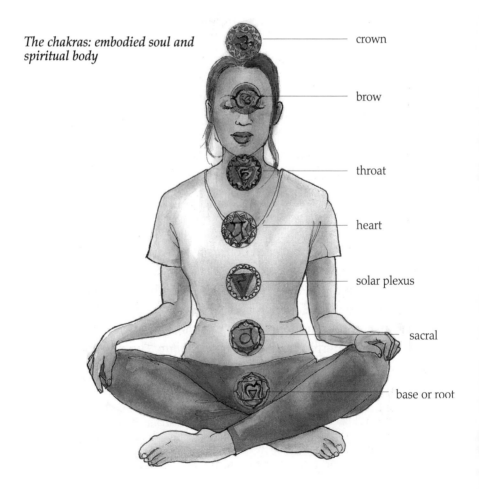

The chakras: embodied soul and spiritual body

crown

brow

throat

heart

solar plexus

sacral

base or root

Table 1

Chakra/ emotional centre	Anatomic structure	Group of organs	Set of emotions/Issues
1st	Body framework	Bones and skeleton, Blood, Immune system	Represents the framework of your life and what moulds your identity: your family, work, religion, community and aspects of your life at an organisation and group level Represents fearfulness and fearlessness, Trust and mistrust, Hope and hopelessness, Dependence and independence
2nd	Pelvis	Sex/reproductive organs, Bladder, Urinary tract, Lower gastrointestinal tract, Lower back	This is about your drives: sex, money, fertility, creativity, Holding on and letting go, Individual within relationship
3rd	Middle abdomen	Gastrointestinal tract, Intestines, Stomach, Pancreas, Kidneys, Liver and Gallbladder	Role in society – acquiring skills and developing competency and confidence Confidence and competence, Self-esteem and power, Fear, sadness, shame
4th	Chest	Heart, Lungs, Breasts	Balance between power and vulnerability Expressing all emotions healthily, Nurturing outward and inwards, Love, passion, intimacy; Midpoint/core of all centres, Oneness in love relationship
5th	Neck/Jaw	Thyroid gland, Throat, Voice box (larynx), Neck vertebrae, Mouth, gums and teeth	Communication, Expression, Asserting yourself in the outside world
6th	Head region	Head, Eyes, Ears, Nose	Knowledge, wisdom and ignorance, Perception and paranoia, Your intellectual self
7th	Beyond body/Whole body	Genes, Connective tissue, Spiritual energy	Purpose, meaning in life; Connection to God/Spirituality; Loneliness and connectedness; Infinite potential and despair and depression

four basic emotions of anger, sadness, happiness and fear may traverse all the chakras.)

I am sharing with you a philosophy that may match a new way of medical thinking. This does not mean that your particular illness or all disease is because of this and that the only way to heal yourself is through your emotions. It is one of many aspects of your complex human functioning. You may or may not connect to this philosophy; it is okay if you choose to discard it. My role is to open some new doors through which you may or may not enter.

It may expand your world view and enable you to internalise yet another approach to improved wellbeing or healing. Do not believe anyone who tells you that the only way is through your chakras or through any one modality. Healing and wellbeing is about the integration of the best of medical science together with authentic healing pathways. And of course, there is so much that is not within your control.

A deep analysis of each emotional centre is beyond the scope of this book. However, the chart below is a simple review of what each emotional centre represents.

Personality types and health

A strong association exists between certain personality types and specific illnesses. You have probably heard and read about type A and type B personalities. Type As tend to be aggressive, driven, impatient and competitive, whereas type Bs are more at ease, in less of a hurry and less ambitious. That type As are more at risk for developing heart disease and ulcers has been commonly accepted by most of mainstream medicine for a long while, and now more information and research is coming to light in this area. Based on the review of your emotions and emotional centres, you can now understand how certain emotions get embedded into certain organs and structures in your body.

Your unique personality, your character traits and emotions may to some extent determine your susceptibility to illness. Once again, this important knowledge is not to make you feel guilty for getting sick, it just highlights how important self-knowledge and especially emotional self-

awareness is in your total health plan (see Chapter 1). For your own quality of life, it is worth improving your negative personality traits as many of
them are within your control.

The most documented research in this field of personality and illness
lies in the area of heart disease and cancer, especially breast cancer. These
are the two most important physical structures found within your fourth
emotional centre – the centre which most expresses the theme of this
chapter: *Embrace and take real care.*

Heart disease and personality
Recent research at Duke University (North Carolina, United States) has
discovered that people who are merely ambitious or driven (Type As)
aren't really the ones at risk for heart disease. According to Duke's
Behavioral Medicine Research Centre, *'Hostility is the real risk factor – people who are angry, abrasive and aggressive'.* The personality type thought to
be associated with coronary disease is now called type H – *hostile and hur-
ried.* They are generally rigid, confrontational and threatening people.
They have an overload of power and an absence of vulnerability. Remember the concept of balancing emotions in expressing power and vulnerability? For optimum health you need a balance of both.

If you have an imbalance between the two or only one side of the
emotion (such as the power here), then this suggests that you may be setting the scene for susceptibility to illness in the organs connected to that
emotional centre.

When you think of this personality type, you immediately imagine a
man. You may think that anger and hostility is not about women's health!
You don't often see women's anger expressed in full force (and if you do,
it is certainly not viewed admiringly!).

In the rapidly changing society in which we live, with the transformation of women into positions of power, you see more and more of what is
referred to as 'masculinisation of emotions' or *the masculinisation of women's
health patterns.* Working women may sometimes become belligerent and
hostile. Worried about being perceived as mediocre or incompetent,
many women go out of their way to prove they are not too emotional or

passive, and can be more aggressive and demanding than any man. This can eventually take its toll on your health.

In addition to the stress that many women experience due to juggling a demanding career with raising a family, there is also the increased susceptibility to illness and especially to those illnesses previously in the domain of men. While you are entitled to the same financial successes and positions of power previously unattainable, you do not want to take on men's disease patterns in addition to your own risks for illness.

Even when hostility is not seen, it does not mean women don't feel it. It may stew inside you, turning into deep bitterness and resentment. And this bitterness can attack a woman's heart in the same way as a man's hostility. This bitterness is another manifestation of deep anger. Just as high levels of expressed anger in the form of hostility are related to heart disease in men, low levels of expressed anger are associated with cardiac disease in women (American Journal of Epidemiology).

While you take action with all the major risk factors for heart disease such as cholesterol and glucose, weight and blood pressure control, exercise, diet and stress management, remember there is huge value in facing and dealing with your negative emotions, especially deep-seated bitterness and resentment.

Breast cancer and personality

Breast cancer, the leading cause of cancer deaths in women, is on the increase worldwide and steadily increasing among black women and younger women in South Africa. So much is as yet unknown about why women develop cancer of the breast. Certain high-risk categories include a strong family history of breast cancer and never having borne children. But generally most medical practitioners are baffled by the scourge of breast cancer. Most often the patient has absolutely no identifiable risk factors. Emotionally you have to face a 'double monster': that of accepting a diagnosis of cancer as well as the possible loss and disfigurement to this structure of your womanhood.

There is no doubt that early detection through screening for breast cancer is the one aspect that *is* within your control. If breast cancer is detected before it has spread to tissues outside the breast, the survival rate is more than 95 percent.

The function of the breast is to nourish and nurture. Your breasts are a symbol of one of your most powerful emotions – love. The breasts are the part of your body to which you closely hold, feed and nurture your loved ones. It is only logical that emotions surrounding love and caring are associated with breast disease – often due to a lack of these emotions when it comes to yourself.

With time, many women slowly but surely sacrifice their own needs in order to take responsibility for everyone else, not only their children but also their partners, older parents and the community. This is lauded and highly valued by society. But there are often internal conflicting emotions (either conscious or subconscious) other than a warm feeling of love.

While taking care of everyone and sacrificing your own needs, the noble self-sacrifice may slowly transform into seeds of resentment. You unknowingly may take on the features of a martyr. A martyr is so focused on self-sacrifice that she needs to repress her own emotions in order to carry everyone else.

Martyrdom is very different from true nurturing. A few studies have demonstrated very strong self-sacrificing qualities in many women with breast cancer. You may take responsibility to the extreme by becoming hyper-responsible for satisfying the needs of those around you. It *is* possible to do too much.

A total imbalance seems to occur between power and vulnerability in your emotional expression, your caring and your relationships. Strangely, in a woman's style of mothering, both extremes are associated with breast cancer – the cold and distant mother as well as the smothering, overprotective mom. You can now identify how these parenting styles reveal the imbalance of the emotions. The overprotective mom has too much external power, combined with a need to control (probably in all areas of her life) whereas the detached mother with excessive vulnerability is withdrawn and internal.

To take this further, some studies have shown that women who accept their cancer with complete stoicism have a worse prognosis than those who express emotions and a healthy fighting spirit. But take this fighting spirit too far into a total self-belief in your power to change and control everything, and the long-term prognosis once again worsens.

You need to be able to love others but also take real care of yourself. You need to feel and express all your emotions fully, including grief and anger, and not hide behind a stoical, brave, martyr front. Be honest and forthright about confronting your negative personality traits and work on them. You need to nurture your internal vulnerability with intimacy in relationships, but especially to make time for yourself; to balance the giving to those around you with the taking care of yourself.

Nurturing

Women know intuitively how to nurture. Regardless of your place in the world or the workplace, there exists within you a deep nurturing instinct. You may have experienced this as a maternal instinct or a great sense of love that surges from a deep source within you. It is an urge to care and comfort. It is a desire to protect and hold close. You may be saying *'Oh no, not me'*. I truly believe as a woman you have it. If you do not feel it, the reason may be that you have had to bury this deep instinct due to your work or circumstance.

But nurturing is not solely the domain of women. Although many men may be discouraged from developing a nurturing capacity whilst growing up, they too have it. Men do, however, express it differently, perhaps as a sense of providing for and protecting others.

But the reality is that at a body level there are differences between the sexes. Together with a woman's ability to carry life and give birth is embedded a natural capacity to nurture. The word nurture comes from the 14th century Latin word for the 'act of nursing' – to nourish and suckle an infant.

The ability to nurse or breastfeed is a physiological process that happens immediately with the birth of your baby. The associated feeling of love and the instinct to take care may be as physiologically integrated within your body and brain as the flow of milk from your breast. This is not to say that at this time in your life there are no issues other than utter love. There are plenty of conflicting emotions including weepiness and utter joy, together with anxiety and even depression (see below). But at a core level the instinct to nurture is there.

To nurture goes way beyond breastfeeding. It means to feed and fill with love and compassion. Your child needs this for his or her very survival. Nurturing is a mother's fierce determination to look after, raise and protect her offspring. You try to give your child the most nourishing food, mental stimulation, guidance, direction and emotional stability. The reason you take care of all your child's needs is to effect the best possible growth and development. The nourishment you give to your child is filled with tenderness, comfort, acknowledgement, security and spiritual sustenance. Without this your child cannot thrive.

Nurturing the nurturer

Without these same things YOU cannot thrive! You need to apply these very same principles to yourself. Yes, you are an adult but the identical nurturing tools that allow your child to thrive are what is needed for yourself. Guess what? You have needs! And the good news is that you are the one that can address most of them. Whatever childhood you may have experienced – whether you received all this nurturing or whether you didn't – as an adult you now have the power to take special care of yourself.

Once again, what is required of you is the balance of power (giving to the outside world) and vulnerability (giving within). For almost all women the scales are completely weighted in the direction of giving outwards. The irony is that you are able so naturally to take care of others, and yet you seldom consider directing it inwards.

But often you feel guilty for having to meet your own needs. You do not feel entitled to rest or pamper or nurture yourself without a little guilt. One of the reasons for this may be that your self-worth and value is based on being completely selfless and generous towards others. What if I told you it is possible to lose your vitality and even get ill if you give too much? I am not saying don't be truly generous and caring, but balance the outward compassion with an inward flow.

The flip side of this totally selfless woman also exists. You certainly know those women who become self-obsessed and narcissistic in the pursuit of pampering, pleasure and body perfection under the guise of nurturing themselves. This is problematic and again you can see the extreme imbalance and lack of true self-awareness. Beneath this shallow exterior there is usually a deep emotional pain and real sense of inadequacy.

What are your needs?

You may not even know what your needs are! While discussing this issue a few years ago during a medical consultation with an extremely fatigued patient, I became aware of a common thread among many of my female patients, that of *being totally unaware of their own needs*. After excluding a medical or psychological cause for her fatigue we discussed her relationships, her busy life as an attorney, her family and community responsibilities. I asked a simple question *'Do you feel your needs are being met?'*

'What needs?' she asked.

I proceeded to make sure she was eating healthily and sleeping well and explained that those were needs, but what about other needs? She was still baffled as she could not identify what she needed. So we continued. *'How about these needs?'* I asked:

✦ Do you feel loved?
✦ Do you receive compassion?
✦ Do you feel appreciated by those around you?
✦ Do you feel heard . . . does your partner listen to what you want to express?
✦ Do you ever have an opportunity to rest when you feel tired ?
✦ Do you make time for your interests and passions – art, gardening, pottery, music etc?
✦ Do you feel you have mental stimulation other than work?
✦ Do you do anything that gives you spiritual sustenance?
✦ Do you ever set aside time that is just for you?

She gave me a blank stare and was aghast. *'Are these my needs?'* she asked? *'I don't really know what your needs are'* I answered. Those listed above are my needs. They may possibly be yours, too. But you are unique and so are your needs. Only you can begin to identify them. All of my needs are not always met and that is okay.

I am conscious of when I am feeling overloaded and try to find ways to meet some of these needs. Whenever possible I try to re-establish the balance of the giving outwards with the giving inwards. There are often times when the scales are tipped heavily in the direction of giving, but it does not always need much to tip back the balance. A massage, a deep undisturbed sleep on a Saturday afternoon, a meditation for 20 minutes in the middle of a busy day, may be enough. And it may keep me feeling resourceful for a while. There are also times where I do not sense that the 'snap' is about to happen until after it has happened: an outburst of anger at my child for a less than serious issue or a flood of tears at a harsh word said to me. Then it takes a bit more than a 20-minute sleep to get back on track. I know I need to take a deeper look at what is really happening, clear through the emotional and mental clutter, make amends, start daily meditations again and implement whatever other steps I need.

On the roller coaster of life as a carer you make sure you bury these needs deep within you and when the unexplained rage and fury or sadness surfaces in unexpected ways and without warning, you do not even know *what you may need* to restore the joy and calm to your life. You know you need to work, you need to care for a family and you have a responsibility to the community at large. You do not feel entitled to need more, until you get ill. The giving outwards without nurturing yourself ultimately manifests in fatigue, burnout, depression and perhaps illness.

This is like an emotionally dwarfed child who may have grown up in an orphanage and never have known the warm morning embrace of his mother and the goodnight hug of his father and the countless acts of affection in between. He would be totally unable to identify his needs. He only knows that he feels horrible inside all the time. He also fails to thrive physically, does not grow properly and may be a sickly child.

A lack of emotional nurturing manifests in physical illness. The human body needs love and nurturing in order to not only thrive but to survive. Take this child and place him in the care of loving human beings, address his most basic emotional needs and watch him flourish.

You too are entitled to flourish. You need to be loved and held and understood. If you can ask for them within a warm loving relationship that exists within your life – do so. But most of the time you need to do it for yourself. And as a carer of others, you need to take time out for self-care. Do it for your health, if nothing else.

You may also suggest that we live in a country with much deprivation, poverty and neediness surrounding us and ask the question *'Is it not selfish to focus too much on your own needs, especially if your own basic needs like food and shelter are already provided for?'* I believe that we live in a country in which everyone has a social responsibility. It should be part of the very fabric of our lives. You and I and all women and men need to give back in whatever way we can – with skills, with money, with caring, with involvement. (That orphan is not just a metaphor. He is one of at least 800 000 children in our country. Giving beyond yourself in acts of loving kindness is also a way to nurture yourself. See Chapter 6.)

Focusing on your needs and nurturing yourself is what fills your inner self so that you can give from a full vessel to those around you. If you cannot fill your cup to the brim, the vessel becomes empty, dry and then eventually cracked. You fill yourself up in order to give of your best to feed your family and serve your community.

How do you nurture yourself?

To answer that question, ask yourself two questions:
1. What do I need in order to take excellent care of myself?
2. How do I go about nurturing myself – what should I do and where do I start to ensure that I am taking the best possible care of my body, my emotions and my whole life?

Time

To nurture yourself you do indeed need time. You are already familiar with Taking charge of your time (from Chapter 1) and interrupting your mantra of *'I have no time'*. Choose simple strategies like the creation of 'white space' in your diary, booking off time just for you, marching at a different pace and establishing time gaps between your activities and commitments. *Taking care* of your time, however, is keeping the appointments with yourself and knowing with what to fill this time.

Time for rest

I classify rest as separate from sleep. Your night's sleep is a basic primary necessity. There are indeed sleep disturbances throughout your life from pregnancy and breastfeeding, sick kids or children with frequent waking, right through to menopausal hot flushes and sleep disorders. Daily frustrations, anxiety and depression may also interfere with your sleep (see Chapter 5). But sleep is not something you should have to schedule into your week planner whereas rest is.

Most women feel entitled to rest only when pregnant or ill. Unfortunately, many women develop frequent complaints or ailments (sometimes subconsciously) in order to feel justified in resting.

Your body is not designed to function on full charge all day. Your unique energy pattern is different from other women but all will experience highs and slumps. Many factors affect this variation and several measures can boost energy levels during the day (see Chapter 5).

Your body sends you fatigue signals. Listen to them. You obviously cannot always respond to each signal. You are in an office for eight hours a day or you are busy with commitments and deadlines or have children in your care. But there are undoubtedly moments when you can respond and rest.

If you do not work but have children to care for, there are many creative ways to get some rest. In South Africa many women employ a caregiver to assist with childminding. If you are privileged to have one, then there is no excuse not to grab a 20-minute gap somewhere in your day. If you cannot afford any babysitting and are not formally working, either rest while the children are at school, while the toddlers take their rest or share responsibilities with a friend and give each other a break occasionally.

Time for pampering

The word pamper means to spoil, indulge, treat, fuss over, coddle and cocoon. You may associate pampering with overindulgence, and there are women who spend far too much time, money and energy on excessive pampering and superficiality. But it is good to intermittently indulge your senses, treat your body and spoil yourself to recreate balance in your life.

Pampering fills a deep internal energy within you. It has the capacity to restore your joy and hope. And guess what? It is good for your body, too. It elicits the release of endorphins and neurotransmitters such as serotonin which lifts your mood, reduces the release of cortisol and adrenalin (the stress hormones) and may even stimulate the outpouring of healing and immune boosting substances within you.

Treat
Treat is a word associated with childhood, especially sweet things on special occasions, holidays, festivals and for good behaviour. Well, bring that word back into your everyday vocabulary! Begin to treat yourself – you deserve it!

On a recent visit to San Francisco to deliver a lecture at a conference, after the hype, the exhaustion and the adrenalin rush of my presentation, I was bewildered when the organiser of the event came up to me and said *'It is now time for "TREAT"!'*. She dragged me a few miles on foot through the undulating streets of San Francisco to a haven of scents, aromas, sounds, beauty, as well as a most gentle healing massage to my aching body. This exquisite pampering store-cum-salon was actually called TREAT! And I understood in that moment that women need pampering and treats just as much as children do in order to thrive.

There are two sorts of pampering – a self-pampering exercise and luxurious pampering at the hands of someone else. Consciously create a pampering ritual for each day. You may not get to do it every day, but even a few times a week will make you feel good and will nourish your sensory system. Your 10 or 20 minute rest during the day may be your pampering time. If you can extend this time, even better. Take off your shoes, lie on your bed or couch, in winter cover your legs with a warm blanket, drink a steaming cup of tea, listen to soothing music, read if you wish, preferably just lie quietly, meditate or do nothing at all.

If you are juggling work and family it will be almost impossible to fit pampering time into the middle of your day. Use the end of the day or even later in the evening to treat yourself. Once the dinner and bedtime ritual is over (if you have that) or right after work or gym, do not rush to attend to chores and accounts. Do something for *you*. Perhaps the best opportunity to enjoy a luxurious pampering ritual is your bathtime, and you do not need to spend much money to transform your bathroom into a haven. Stimulate all your senses by acquiring fragrant soaps, bath oils and candles. Different aromatherapy oils or fragrances are thought to have different effects. Lavender and rosemary are calming, lemon grass and basil are balancing, whereas vanilla and cinnamon are energising. Awaken your sense of sound with meditative relaxing music and perhaps even take a mug of your favourite cinnamon or exotic fruit tea or even a steaming mug of hot chocolate to enthuse your sense of taste. Bask in the feel, the sounds, the flavours, the warmth, the fragrances and the mood.

To be treated to a pampering session at the hands of someone else is wonderful. If you can afford to spoil yourself with a regular massage or a facial by a professional, you will be doing wonders to your back, your feet, your hands, your face or your whole body. But the effects will not only be a good feeling through your skin and muscles. Healing will also take place.

If you cannot afford such a luxury, why not take turns with your partner by giving each other a healing massage every few weeks? Turn on some soothing music, light a candle and all you need buy is a small amount of massage oil. You may choose to be the recipient or provider of the massage with no strings attached for the therapeutic benefits, or to indulge in this massage as a prelude to greater intimacy. If you do not have a partner, why not suggest to your friends or office mates that they give you a voucher for a massage as a birthday present rather than more coffee mugs or hand cream

The basic goal of massage therapy is to help the body heal itself and to increase health and wellbeing. Touch is the core ingredient of massage therapy. Areas of tension within the skin and muscles are relieved. Touch also conveys a sense of caring, an important component in the healing. Massage improves your circulation, which increases your blood flow, bringing fresh oxygen to body tissues. This can assist with the elimination of waste products such as lactic acid from muscle use, speed healing after injury, and enhance recovery from disease. Other benefits may be enhanced immunity, better lymph drainage, a soothed nervous system, improved muscle and skin tone and digestion, and a decrease in your blood pressure due to the relaxation response. It may also help relieve acute or chronic pain. Different massage techniques have been developed and integrated into many health systems in both mainstream and complementary medicine.

Time for 'Time outs'

Despite your numerous demands, you have the control to say 'time out guys' *mainly to yourself*. I propose that you take a 'time out' at least once a week, at the very least, 30 minutes to an hour a week for time out.

It is your appointment with yourself – the white space that you have booked in your week planner. I recommend that your time out is often spent on your own. At times you may choose to spend it with your partner or with girl friends. You wither in isolation; you blossom with nourishing friendships. You need your female friendships in the good times and especially the bad times. Nurture these friendships but remember to spend your special time with those friends who energise and do not drain you further.

What you choose to do in that time is anything that makes your heart sing. The pampering massage or manicure is an ideal 'time out' exercise. But there are many other ways to nurture this time. Turn it into a adventurous pursuit of your interests or passions.

'Time out' with recreation

The conventional wisdom of recreation seems to describe a whole host of activities for people who have very little to do: baking, sewing, photography, painting, crafts and the like. This could not be further from the truth. Recreation comes from the word to recreate. Through creative endeavours such as painting, pottery or gardening you literally recreate your life force, your energy, your joy. You are able to ignite your passions. But recreation need not only be 'creative' exercises. It can be anything that allows you to *recreate* your vitality within.

Spend a period of time in a beautiful garden, go to a movie or theatre or concert, a dance class, a session of yoga, a half-hour in a book store or a coffee shop. The list is endless.

This time out allows you to begin to follow your heart. You may not even know what your interests are (they may be deeply buried together with your needs). So wander through an art supplies or photography shop, a florist or a vintage décor store, and begin to discover each week what interests you.

If it is looking at clothes in a mall, that's okay, although I suspect that after a while clothes shopping becomes a draining experience for many women and I would advise against using time out each week to shop for clothes (as then it becomes toiletries and then food; do grocery shopping online and save yourself an extra hour at least per week!).

You may love cooking or baking. Many women find it very relaxing and fulfilling and do not get to prepare much more than basic family meals. So use this hour once a week to cook up a storm. Once again turn on beautiful music, ignite your senses and savour the aromas, the sounds and the flavours coming out of your kitchen. Let this time out become a time to discover your passions.

'Time out' with spiritual pursuits

You may choose to fill your time out with spiritual pursuits. This may include spending the half-hour in prayer or in meditation. If you have already set aside time each day for prayer or meditation or introspection (see Chapter 6), then this weekly pursuit may be a time to read and study further. You should be already spending some time exercising in your week so for this half-hour choose a more 'mind-spirit-body' modality such as yoga or t'ai chi, if this appeals to you.

There is yet one more suggestion for this time out each week. I call it a spiritual pursuit, you may choose to call it social responsibility.

Acts of loving kindness seem to be a nurturing of others rather than a self-nurturing. I believe that the act of giving to those beyond your immediate family, to those in need materially or financially, but more important, emotionally, are deeds that nurture your own soul. How do you do this? Visit the local senior citizens or frail care home and just sit with one or two lonely people for a few moments, perhaps reading to someone with impaired vision or listening to a lonely individual's story. Go to a shelter for abandoned or abused children or HIV orphans and simply participate in a puzzle activity. Or volunteer your services even once-off to help with meals to the destitute. Even better, do this on a weekend and take one of your children with you. (You obviously need to speak to the authorities or social workers at the institution beforehand.)

There are numerous opportunities everywhere, but especially in this country, to do small acts of loving kindness. People may scoff at such ideas as self-righteous or too small to make a difference. If you are the CEO of a company and can do big things with big money in the realm of social responsibility then do it! But if you are working, juggling a family and attempting to raise children or grandchildren who care, take a half-hour, meet with a lonely, aged woman, let your child read a story or listen to hers, and you will be nurturing at least three souls all at once.

Self-acceptance

This is the second prerequisite for taking excellent care of yourself. You cannot take care of anything without valuing it highly, but I cannot just instruct you to acknowledge, respect and value yourself. It is not so simple. But I also think that it need not be so complicated. Sure, you may have had a difficult childhood with major traumas or you have been abandoned or jilted many times. Or you may have none of the above but still do not feel good about yourself. Self-acceptance is undoubtedly an area that improves with effective psychotherapy and counselling and you may have to go through or continue to go through a process with a therapist while dealing with many life issues.

But self-acceptance can to a large extent be developed on your own. It does not depend on you being the most successful businesswoman, outstanding mother or physically exquisite. It depends on starting to make a head decision (see Chapter 1) to acknowledge and appreciate yourself and then moving into a 'heart' space where you can begin to feel this.

Three aspects of being a woman affect your self-acceptance: *I am beautiful, I am valuable, I am good enough*. Begin to develop these areas by altering your belief patterns (see Take charge of your perceptions in Chapter 1) by feeding your head and your heart new information.

I am beautiful

Every woman is beautiful. You may look in the mirror and see blemishes and many imperfections. You may see ageing. You may hate your nose or your profile or your overweight body and self-loathing follows.

If you are able for a moment to look past those few things and truly take a real good look at yourself, you may begin to reach a sense of self-acceptance. A popular song by Christina Aguilera has the words *'I am beautiful no matter what they say . . . and life can't bring me down'*. These words need to be your new motto.

When I say I believe that every woman is beautiful, I am not only referring to a deep untapped internal kindness and warmth, I mean external beauty, too. If you can look beyond your faults and imperfections, you will begin to see some areas of light – beautiful eyes or a defined jawline or lovely skin or a fantastic smile. Decide that it is time to make peace with your body and your face with all its imperfections and faults. And begin to appreciate the enormous gift of your physical self. Begin to use your face (with its faults and blemishes). The power of a smile does not just enhance your beauty but has the power to lift someone else's flagging spirits.

I am valuable

You have value in the workplace, in your home and with your friends. It is so easy to doubt your self-worth. Sure, you have weaknesses like everyone else, but also strengths.

Even if you're in a bumpy relationship or an unfulfilling job, you *are* valuable. If you cannot see your significance, begin to dig beneath the surface and truly uncover your value. Say it to yourself, say it to your children, say it to your partner: *'I am valuable'*. Walk tall and behave like a valued person, and you *will* begin to feel it. You have a role or many roles to play which have immense value (not always measurable by you!).

Being valuable does not read *'I am precious'*, meaning *'I need to be put on a pedestal, treat me with greater respect than other women because I have a perfect figure or enormous bank balance'*. All women deserve respect and consideration.

I am good enough

Self-acceptance also means believing '*I am good enough*'. This is different from '*I am valuable*'. This concept of good enough may go against much of the culture we live in. Most of the self-help and enrichment manuals are preaching achievement, improvement and change. Of course, there is always room for personal progress but the media and the experts keep telling you how to change yourself into something other than what you are. Telling you that '*Who you are is not enough. Do more to be a better mother, a better executive, a better soul. Do more, become more*'. Stop for a moment and say '*I am good enough*'.

If your intention is to CHANGE who you are, you will probably fail. If your intention is to BECOME who you truly are, you cannot help but live a balanced, meaningful life. The things you can change are your perceptions, your choices, your behaviours and your actions, but not *you*.

But what is good enough? If you say that, you need to be absolutely honest. It doesn't mean mediocre, second-rate, negligent or reckless. Good enough means responsible, committed, caring and productive.

The good enough mother does not say '*I have now had enough of this – I will feed the kids four nights a week only and cut the time I spend with them in half*'. A good enough mother is a parent who is responsible in her parenting role, is present as much as possible, gives warmth and strength and direction from within her own authentic warmth and strength. She is not detached and cold and selfish. But she need not be mothering in a way that smothers, that does not allow any space for herself or space for her child to breath on his or her own. Smothering children is destructive. Children need security and boundaries between themselves and their parents, together with love and warmth. A good enough mother creates this balance of outward flow with inward flow, of love with restraint.

The drive of the 21st century, especially for women, is on 'getting ahead', 'moving up the ladder', 'doing it all' and 'having it all'. You *can* be good enough in the workplace, too. That does not mean that you cannot achieve excellence. Good enough means you do not need to go beyond your personal boundaries in order to prove yourself and please others. You do need to fulfil performance criteria and give of your best but you do not need to behave in a way or be what you are not in order to please or demand authority. You need not become aggressive and hostile or demeaning and servile.

What has this got to do with your health? By never feeling good enough you set up a pattern of living a life where your internal self and your external behaviour are completely unmatched. You cannot fool your body. This disconnection between what you are truly feeling and thinking and what you are portraying to the world is a betrayal of your body. Your body picks up this imbalance and manifests stress, fatigue, exhaustion and compromise of your immunity (see Chapter 1 Authenticity).

Take care of your emotions

Since the essence of nurturing is expressed at an emotional level, this is the best place to start taking care of yourself. You now have a deeper understanding of how emotions are represented in your physical body. You have also embraced the concept of your fourth emotional centre. This area literally embodies nurturing. It houses your heart, your breasts and your deepest emotion – love. You understand that for the good of your health, it is essential to take care of your emotional self, too.

If you experience excessive anger or you feel quite sad most of the time or even if you just require some clarity and insight into your emotions, you may require the help of a professional.

It is completely normal to feel most emotions throughout your day or your week. If something upsets you or pleases you, you respond with a feeling. An essential part of being alive is the surfacing of feelings which you experience as good or bad. There are constant triggers to set off your emotions. What you do with them matters to your health. You are entitled to feel angry when someone lets you down, pleased when it works out or sad when you have a disappointment. Generally you feel it and after a while move on. (*Remember emotion means 'to move', to go forward.*) You need to be on alert when you find yourself stuck in the emotion and cannot move on.

Or you may find that the unpleasant feelings are with you most of the time. The anger may stew inside you or you find yourself waking up feeling miserable. It would help to exercise (see Chapter 4) and implement a meditation programme (see Chapter 5) but you may need more than this. If you feel weepy most of the day and then go to bed still feeling low and sleep poorly, you should seek professional help. You do not need to feel so bad, and there is no shame in seeking out help. Part of being alive may involve times of imbalance.

Let's take a look at two powerful healing emotions: love and passion.

Love
The old cliché 'Love makes the world go round' has profound relevance to your health. Both nurturing and being nurtured are life-enhancing. Much scientific evidence exists and continues to grow in medical literature on the health-damaging consequences of loneliness and isolation and the life-enhancing power of love and intimacy. Some of this research reveals that those with the least emotional support double their premature death rate. Those who were the loneliest and most isolated had almost four times the risk of dying prematurely. The first of this research, conducted by Professor David Spiegel of Stanford University in the late 1980s, demonstrated that even a few weeks of strong, social support can affect recurrence and survival from cancer many years later. Intimacy and loving bonds lead to healing whereas isolation and loneliness lead to suffering and illness.

This philosophy is the core of Dr Dean Ornish's remarkable heart disease 'reversal' centres in the United States. Patients are subjected to stringent diet and exercise programmes, but the most important ingredient in the programme is dealing with emotions, especially love. Dr Ornish describes how in the healing of all illnesses, loving and intimate bonds are more powerful healing factors than drugs, genetics, surgery, diet or exercise.

You may be thinking: *'What if I do not have a loving partner or family, does that mean I may get ill or not heal?'* I believe that the power of love is undeniably healing, but it is one of numerous factors. And if you do not receive this love within your immediate family, firstly continue to give out love and secondly go out and find a support group that can provide the safety, the warmth, the listening and the unconditional support that is vital to your health. It may be a group of close women friends, a regular coffee or lunch team or a support group of people in the same situation or life stage as you.

Passion

Passion is a very powerful and healing emotion. It is a tugging of your heart. It is being intimate with your longings and desires. Living passionately gives meaning to your life. The synergy between passion and a purpose fires up your immune system producing active substances to ward off illness, mop up damaged cells and augment the body's healing and defences. To live with passion is to open yourself to all the complexities of life, to choose to live to the fullest.

In my work with cancer and other life-threatening conditions, it is clear that many people cope more easily with these challenges if they recognise that life has a deep sense of meaning. There is much documented medical research demonstrating the connection between passion, purpose and physical healing. An important area of this research lies in the field of PNI (psychoneuroimmunology). This is an interesting subject studying the pathways between thoughts, the mind, neurological (nervous system) and immunity.

Amazingly physical healing does take place as a direct result of the passion and purpose with which you live. It builds a reservoir of physical and emotional power enabling you to withstand your stresses and sorrows. You need to search for what gives your life meaning and what ignites your passion.

Take care of your body

Your physical body essentially operates independently of your personal attention and care. Your heart beats, your lungs supply oxygen, your digestion moves, your hormones and enzymes are released, your immunity destroys invaders, your nerves relay messages, your cells communicate with one another and millions of complicated processes occur without your knowledge or intervention. The most awe-inspiring aspect of your body is its inherent design to continuously restore balance and harmony within. Even when illness is present, there is so much that is still performing efficiently.

Notwithstanding this automatic control, there are personal choices that you make that either damage or enhance this dynamic configuration. You have the choice to take excellent care of your body.

The most basic element in nurturing your physical body is how you nourish it. Good nutrition is essential. Food is the fuel that drives most of the processes, including healing and renewal. (Follow the 10 basic principles outlined in Chapter 3.)

Undoubtedly beginning an exercise programme or improving your current exercise plan is the single most important facet in maintaining and nurturing your body. Simply by exerting yourself and moving about, you can transform nearly every part of your body and mind. The physical benefits are numerous and there are also marked mental and emotional health gains. It is as simple as that, a dynamic lifestyle which includes exercise is the cornerstone of taking care of your body (see Chapter 4). It is not all about cardio training. Remember as you age to include flexibility and strength training, too, to ensure strong bones, muscles and skin.

Make sure your sleep hygiene is a priority in taking care of your body. Good quality sleep and adequate rest is necessary for your brain and nervous system to carry out its central role. All vital processes throughout your body have peaks and troughs and many are optimised by the smooth flow of your circadian rhythm – your 24-hour body clock. This cycle depends on quality sleep to maintain itself. Sleep has an enormous restorative capacity (see Chapter 5).

From your 'take charge' strategy (see Chapter 1) you have become empowered to make decisions and be proactive about your body. You now move to the 'take care' strategy where you embrace and begin to truly nurture your physical body. It is hoped you now have a sense of what you need to take real good care; setting aside some time for pampering, for rest, for recreation, for stress release, for passion as well as acknowledging your beauty and your value as a woman, a mother and a person with a contribution to make.

This remarkable physical structure houses the real YOU – your unique personality, your independent thinking, your feelings and your spirit. As a woman your body, too, has the power to create, hold and carry life. Do not dismiss your physical self as fat or old or only bodily. Look after it, appreciate it, pamper it, celebrate and enjoy it.

Take care of your beauty

For a doctor involved with the treatment and prevention of real disease, is it not superficial of me to urge you to take care of your beauty? As a woman myself and working with many women in healthcare, there is no doubt that all women want to look and feel in some way beautiful. And so they should. All women are indeed beautiful and this needs to be nurtured and taken care of.

I have seen breast cancer patients in the midst of deeply traumatic surgery, chemotherapy and life crises. Whether these women are 30 and in their gorgeous prime or 80 in their autumn years, they still yearn to maintain a sense of femininity and beauty. The loss or disfigurement of a breast has absolutely nothing to do with vanity and superficiality. It is a deep pain due to an assault on a woman's essential power, femininity and beauty. I encourage these women to do all that may be needed to restore this sense of feeling beautiful.

When addressing the concept of beauty it is vital to be honest and realistic. You are entitled to be the most beautiful woman you can be and to nurture this beauty throughout your life. But it is essential to maintain a balanced approach to your external beauty and self-care. Beauty is one very important aspect of a woman that can easily become a source of great anguish and obsession. You often confuse physical beauty with happiness and fulfillment.

It is indeed wonderful to look and feel good inside and out. But for many women much of the focus on physical beauty sets up several negative life patterns. These include striving for perfection, feelings of inadequacy, overvaluing youthfulness, attempting to deny ageing, self-loathing and developing a 'mannequin-like' existence by investing so much energy in maintaining a façade.

Today there is indeed an overlap between beauty and health. There is a blurring of the boundaries for many reasons, one of which is very interesting: neither ideal beauty nor perfect health is attainable. Yet there is a constant pursuit of a magic approach that will enable you to reach the fountain of youth and beauty or the well of total health and immortality. In the pursuit of eternal youth, wrinkle-free skin and perfect features, many women are in fact searching for elusive happiness and fulfillment. In the same way that health is so much more than your physical body structure, beauty is much more than physical proportion.

Having said that, it is indeed essential firstly to take care of your skin. Your skin is the largest of all your body organs and the one of which you are most aware. It has many important functions other than making you glow!

The skin acts as a barrier preventing the entry of chemicals, particles and organisms such as bacteria into the body. The skin also maintains a balanced internal environment by preventing the loss of water and minerals. It maintains temperature regulation, controls sensation and the synthesis of vitamin D.

The elastic tissue in the skin provides resilience although elasticity does decrease with age, causing skin to wrinkle.

For great care of your skin you need a good, healthy, balanced diet with lots of fresh fruits and vegetables, seven to eight glasses of water a day, seven to eight hours of sleep a night, exercise in fresh air and most importantly a daily beauty regime. If you can afford to pamper yourself with regular facial skin treatments and best quality beauty products, indulge yourself. But you do not need hundreds of fancy products to maintain a good skin.

As a guideline, your skin needs two staples: cleanser and moisturiser. Some experts say that toning is essential. Many dermatologists suggest that it is unnecessary and may even cause extra drying to already dry skin. Other products might include exfoliators and eye cream. Cleansing is the first step in caring for your skin. Throughout the day, sweat, grease, dust, stale make-up, dirt and bacteria tends to collect on your skin and needs to be removed.

Soap and water do tend to remove the impurities but are incapable of removing make-up completely, hence proper cleansing is required with a cream or gel or water-based product. It need not be expensive, but should match your skin type. Toning is thought to remove the greasiness remaining from cleansing preparations, closes open pores and refines your skin giving it a smooth clean texture. All skin types need some type of moisturising. Once again they should be matched to your skin type; young oily skin does not need a rich cream as does an ageing, drier type. The best choice of a moisturiser is that which has a sun protection factor of at least 15!

In our beautiful country with its cobalt blue African skies and warm sunshine, remember to protect your skin, especially your face. The most important product in your beauty care 'war chest' is a good sunscreen. This can be part of your moisturiser or a separate product, if you prefer. You should use this sunblock daily throughout the year. Protecting the skin from the sun needs to be an essential part of your daily skin care routine. Most of the UV light from the sun falls in two main wavelength bands: UVA and UVB. UVA ages the skin; the rays travel far into the skin and cause free-radical damage. These UVAs are responsible for cancers and certain skin sensitive reactions. UVBs burn and brown the skin (by triggering the pigment melanin) and can cause skin cancer. The UVB rays are even stronger than the UVA rays.

Although the damage does not show up immediately, excess sun can be the skin's worst enemy. It is the main cause of premature ageing of your skin. The greater the sun exposure, the faster the damage. This is not only true for white or fair-skinned women. The top layer of all skin has specialised pigment producing cells. These are called melanocytes and produce and contain melanin granules. Melanin is the substance that creates pigment and colour in your skin. It also offers some protection from the sun; the more melanin the better the protection. Although darker skin contains many more melanocytes and much more protection in the form of melanin, there is still potential for damage.

Long-term exposure to the sun is one of the major causes of wrinkles, the other being progressive ageing. As the elastic collagen fibres in the skin weaken, the skin begins to sag. From the age of about 25, regular facial massage may help to preserve some of the elasticity and resilience of the skin by improving the circulation of blood to its surface. Of the many available products promising to reduce wrinkles, some may work, and although some are endorsed by dermatologists and promise a scientific approach, reversing the wrinkles with creams has not been proven by standardised clinical medical trials. There are other ways to remove wrinkles, like the injection of botox and plastic surgical methods. But the choice to undergo plastic surgery for cosmetic reasons is a very personal one. You need to be fully informed of all the possible complications and benefits before taking a decision on plastic surgery. You also need to be realistic about your expectations and your reasons for embarking on this route.

What is real beauty?
It is unquestionably a physical appearance, the proportion of facial features, complexion and quality of skin that contributes to real beauty. There are many beauty therapists, products and make-up that may boost your physical appearance. Indulge yourself and enhance your loveliness.

But beauty is so much more. It is a depth of character, expression of your real self, a unique personality, compassion and caring! Part of the problem of being dissatisfied with who you are and how you look may be due to a denial of your real worth. Inner beauty is a quality so naturally and inherently a deep part of you. The way to enhance this beauty is by pampering yourself. But it is also through quiet introspective methods to connect and grow your spiritual muscle, live with passion and generate an internal energy (see Chapter 6). You need to ignite your own internal light.

The late Dr Elizabeth Kubler-Ross, a remarkable medical doctor and author, famous for her work on the process of dying, compares you to a pane of magnificent stained glass on show in a cathedral, a synagogue, a temple or mosque. When the sun is up, it shines through the magnificent pane of glass and your beauty is apparent. But when the sun goes down, when life gets rough with pain, with illness and suffering unless the light, that internal fire is turned on within, the beauty and vitality is no longer apparent.

Take care of your sexuality

In my clinical experience, many patients, especially married women from different walks of life, shared one extremely interesting feature. They complained of a lack of interest in sex. I was sure that my female practice was an unrepresentative sample of the population, but as I continued to investigate this issue, I realised that a lot the hype and talk about sex was in fact just that: hype and talk.

You can find piles of women's publications bursting with information on sex – weird and wonderful positions, sex tools and multiple orgasms. These articles may help you but more often instead of giving you the confidence to trust yourself and your deep instinctual impulses, they encourage you to stand back from your body and judge how to do it better!

This lack of libido may be due to numerous factors. A lack of libido is seldom an isolated single feature. It may arise from feelings of inadequacy and poor self-esteem, it may be pure exhaustion from work, a lack of sleep or family demands. It may be rooted in childhood traumas, side effects of medication, stress, gynaecological issues or depression.

Women are also often encouraged to repress their sexuality to preserve their vulnerability and therefore may subconsciously inhibit their own libido.

But just as exercise, healthy nutrition and stress management are cornerstones of wellbeing, so too is nurturing your sexuality a vital ingredient of a healthy lifestyle. *The two most common causes of poor libido are the oral contraceptive pill and Prozac.* If you are on one or both of these medications and you have a very low libido (if it concerns you and your partner), please discuss possible alternatives with your doctor.

What many women fail to understand is that their sexuality needs to be nurtured and cared for. The reality is quite different from the media hype. Sure, there are women with bold libidos who enjoy quick and spontaneous sex. In my experience these women are usually unattached and without too many domestic responsibilities. For the most part, arousal in women is not usually a quick, spontaneous process. Effort is required to nurture your sexual energy. It demands communication, relationship building, personal growth and a willingness to express your vulnerability.

It is essential that as a woman you become vigilant about *safe sex*. It is great if you are able to communicate openly with your partner, but even if you cannot, you need to be extremely assertive about insisting on safe sex practices. The use of condoms are essential, especially if you do not have a monogamous relationship.

Your sexuality is not exclusively defined by the sex act. It is a deep, internal, creative energy. It is the energy from which your children are made. This creativity has the potential as well to build your intimate relationship and fuel you in all areas of your life; in areas of art and literature and expressions of love. Sexuality itself possesses both a body and a soul, a physical and a spiritual dimension. The sexual urge is a need to unite with another. Sexuality is this union, this merging into oneness. It is a magnificent force that needs to be honoured and expressed healthily.

You may have sexual interactions that are 'okay' but do not leave you feeling deeply satisfied. This is a common complaint of women. What you may not realise is that in order to experience the sexual act in all its power, you need to expose and experience your vulnerability in all its intensity. You need to 'let go' completely to experience the highest peaks. The concept of intimacy is a celebration of your vulnerability. It touches the softest, most private and fragile part of you. It is for this reason that your relationship must be safe in order to experience true intimacy. Most women desire true intimacy and closeness. But many are afraid to let go of control. Remaining in control and experiencing a multiple orgasm (okay, even a single orgasm!) are mutually exclusive. You cannot do both at the same time. This inability to let go completely makes it impossible to ever experience true satisfaction. The illusion of intimacy leaves you with a feeling of emptiness instead of pure bliss.

If there are any deep-seated emotional scars from childhood or serious unresolved relationship problems or a medical cause for a flagging libido, please do seek help. If none of these issues exist, then the steps needed to nurture your sexuality are quite simple.

If you get turned on quite quickly when your longstanding partner simply suggests its time for bed, you are one of those lucky gals. Generally, most women do not get aroused in the same way as a man. Many men experience a quick and instant turn-on, possibly related to a brief touch or the sight of you in your underwear. The sight of your man in his boxers may do it for you. If so, you are one of fortunate ladies (once again). Most women, however, process arousal in a much more complex way. It takes quite a bit of warmth and kindness from your man or a bit of self-pampering to do it. It often involves thinking about sex and all it involves. Women are said to process through their heads first. A useful tip is to use mind-body techniques. Mind-body methods in the realm of sexuality means 'fantasy' – not necessarily about someone else. But start fantasising earlier in the day, or in the bath. Consciously think more about sex during the day.

Often if you are not really in the mood but you begin the journey of foreplay and ask your partner for a slower process, you will reach the point of excitement with a bit of time. Women generally go through the stages of sexual arousal much more slowly than men. The four stages are called *excitement, plateau, orgasm and resolution*. A man may go through all four phases before his partner has even moved out of phase one (i.e. she is hardly aroused yet!). By understanding this, as well as the fact that it may take a long time of clitoral stimulation to achieve orgasm, both you and your partner could reach new levels of satisfaction. Achieving orgasm is desirable and extremely pleasurable but for many women is not essential each and every time. Also, do not believe all that you read: only 20 per cent of women can achieve orgasm through intercourse alone. The other 80 per cent require clitoral stimulation and for some women it takes a very long time. But the good news is that as you increase the frequency of achieving orgasm, it begins to take a shorter period of time to reach it. What you may not know is that there are side effects of medication that interfere with your sexual experience. One of the side effects of Prozac is an extremely protracted time to reach orgasm or a total inhibition of orgasm for both men and women.

What helps enormously to enhance your libido and sexual experience is for you to take charge. You be the one to initiate sex. This is a big turn-on for your partner and you. It expresses great sexual confidence. And even if you do not feel so confident to start, try it and you will slowly develop sexual self-confidence. Taking a pampering bath with beautiful products, candles and body oils is always a good idea to get you in the mood. Put on great underwear and you initiate the course of action.

To reclaim your sexual energy and become sexually confident and self-assured, you need to embrace it and truly nurture it. You need to apply all the principles already mentioned in this chapter: self-acceptance, self-love, identifying your needs, pampering yourself and balancing external action with internal vulnerability.

Emotions and sex

The subject of boosting your sexuality and enhancing your libido is really interesting from the perspective of emotional health. You may think of sex as purely physical: there is the arousal of sexual organs and then intimate physical contact. But in reality it is a hugely emotional experience (especially for women).

It is a sensory experience that is enmeshed in *feelings*. There is certainly a feeling of lust and it is hoped you have a feeling of love which translates into a warm body feeling and a desire for physical and emotional closeness. You then feel further joy and passion. Your feelings of bliss become transmitted into waves of physical arousal, with more blood flowing into your vaginal tissue which causes the tingling sensation.

Your emotional feelings of pleasure and excitement are conveyed to your clitoris and other erogenous zones. These waves of excitement take you slowly into the further stages and heights of sexual arousal. There is a flow from the emotional to the physical. If this is allowed to surge, it is wonderful.

However, there are many things that interrupt this sexual current. Most commonly it does not even get going from the outset (hence the poor libido). The point at which many women get stuck is being unable to move from the stage of wanting warmth and closeness to being aroused to the point of desiring real excitement and exhilaration (with or without orgasm).

Many of the reasons for this are rooted in the emotional process. Extraneous factors such as utter exhaustion, depression, medications and many other causes already mentioned may interrupt this 'emotion to

78

arousal process', but in the overwhelming majority of circumstances it is due to an imbalance in the power/vulnerability ratio. The concept of balancing your power with your vulnerability is so magnificently seen in the sexual act. Begin to find this power within you by:

+ Initiating sex.
+ Expressing your needs to your partner and experimenting to find what works.
+ Choosing how and where you are together.
+ Guiding the pace of the experience. For example, if you do not yet feel fully turned on, request your partner to slow down or try something else.

To move into an ecstatic desire for fulfilment, you need to feel and express your power as a woman. A woman who feels controlled or repressed or the need to be submissive during the sex act will never experience the heights of female sexual satisfaction.

BUT at the very height of your sexual confidence and power (and maybe even some control) you need to do the exact opposite in order to reach fulfilment, both in terms of an orgasm and/or the depths of intimacy. You need to let go completely and express the deepest core of your vulnerability. As long as you keep holding on, you cannot reach the point of ecstasy.

To express the vulnerability within you:

+ Get to know and love your body.
+ Appreciate the pleasure you are able to experience.
+ Use visualisation, during the day, at any time – imagine yourself letting go into the realm of exhilarating pleasure.
+ Use visualisation during the sexual experience – focus on the *letting go*. Visualise the waves of arousal and the act of 'letting go of all the control'.

It seems like an impossibility but you need to have both intense power and extreme vulnerability at the very same time. Moments of real meaning are described as 'losing yourself'. You lose yourself into utter joy or laughter or in prayer. So, too, in the sexual act through the losing of yourself into your vulnerability, the boundaries dissolve. And through the losing, you actually are *finding* yourself and the intimacy and satisfaction you so greatly desire.

G-Spot

The clitoris is not the only source of pleasure. The G-spot is a small area of erogenous tissue inside the front wall of the vagina, which responds to stimulation. Something that few men (and women themselves) do not know is that it cannot be felt or located when unaroused. It may feel too sensitive or uncomfortable before you are aroused. With arousal it becomes extremely sensitive and pleasurable. Very few women can actually experience orgasm from stimulation of the G-spot alone and require clitoral stimulation as well, but it is certainly a highly erogenous area which feels deeply pleasurable.

Sex and your health

What is clearly apparent is that sex is pleasurable and deeply sustaining in a relationship. Less apparent is it's potent effect on health and immunity. Researchers have revealed how a regular sex life helps ward off illness by boosting the immune system. Doctors have discovered that the level of 'natural killer cells' and 'antibodies' that fight infection is much higher in couples who make love regularly. Regular lovemakers are likely to experience far fewer colds, viruses and 'flu.

Cortisol, a powerful stress hormone, is suppressed during sexual arousal, making sexual activity a great stress buster. A frequent outpouring of the 'feel-good' factors, including endorphins, lifts depression, blunts anxiety and leaves you with a deep sense of wellbeing.

Lovemaking is good for fitness, too. A typical bout of lovemaking is equivalent to sprinting 200 metres. It is demanding on the body, raising your blood pressure, pulse and breathing rate. Every part of your body plays some role in the sexual act.

Starting from the top of your head, sexual arousal sparks off the release of neurotransmitters (chemical messengers) in the brain which begin to stimulate the pituitary gland. This is the command centre for lovemaking. The pituitary also sends messages to your adrenal gland which starts to produce sex hormones and within seconds releases adrenalin which increases heart rate, blood pressure and rapid breathing. More blood is diverted to your genitals to prepare them for the forthcoming activity. The quick gasps of lovemaking indicate the level of exertion taking place in the lungs. Muscle tension increases and your skin's sensitivity heightens, particularly in the erogenous zones.

The gastric acid secretion is increased during lovemaking, possibly as a side effect of the adrenalin surge. This is responsible for the increase in appetite after sex. After orgasm (as in after the sprint) muscle tension relaxes immediately, heartbeat returns to normal and the pituitary switches off the cascade of hormones. The benefits and healing effects then all come into play.

The process of embracing, nurturing and taking care of yourself takes you to the verse expressed by the prophet Ezekiel a few thousand years ago: '*I will remove your heart of stone and give you a heart of flesh*'. Such a heart allows not only your blood but also your emotions to flow forth with health and vitality.

Practical Plan ✦

✦
Month 2:
Take care
✦

BY NOW YOU have implemented the Empower phase of your Personal Health Action Plan and have identified any risk factors for illness, recognised what disease screening is necessary for this stage of your life, begun to take charge of your body and your personal health, documented your physical parameters and implemented some positive lifestyle habits. This month is the opportunity to take excellent CARE of yourself and your health.

✦
Week 1:
Get out of your head and into your heart!
✦

To implement excellent self-care this week, begin by moving out of your head for a while. This head space is indeed the place that thinks, but it is also the space in which you rationalise, you detach, you bargain and you cut off from feelings. The head is the space in which all your self-talk happens.

During this week there will be many questions to ask and not many answers or plans of action offered. Do not worry because you will begin lots of action next week and the months that follow!

The reason for all these questions is that in order to take care of and nurture yourself, you need a great deal of self-awareness. The more you understand about yourself and your blind spots, the more you can begin to identify what requires extra care.

Check your heart

This is the week for a serious and honest appraisal of your emotions. The way to do this is with a CARDIAC check from within your heart. It is hoped you took care of the blood pressure, cholesterol and physical cardiac requirements last month.

The cardiac check assists you in examining your six emotions – their healing or damaging effects and the overload and imbalances in your emotional health.

C   Contentment
A   Anger
R   Resentment
D   Depression
I   Intimacy
A   Anxiety
C   Courage

Take a check this week and continue to be cardiac aware:
1. Am I *Content* with my life? Is their happiness within?
    Contentment does not require a perfect stress-free,
    pain-free life. It is an ability to reach an acceptance
    and appreciation of what you have.
2. Am I carrying and expressing excessive *Anger*? Do I
    manifest any unnecessary hostility?
3. Is *Resentment* deeply buried beneath the surface? This
    stewing resentment is not good for your heart, your
    breasts and your body. There is no value in being a
    martyr. Can you begin to let it go? Forgiveness heals.
4. Am I in any way suffering from features of *Depression*?
    (see page 283) This is the week to seek help.
5. Do I experience healthy *Intimacy*? Do I nurture my
    loving relationships? Can I give and receive love?
6. Is my life filled with excessive *Anxiety*? This is the
    week to confront fears and worries and examine
    whether the anxiety is part of a depression.
7. Do I have *Courage*? Courage is a French derivative for
    the word heart. This is the week to augment your
    courage: your courage to express who you are in the
    world, the courage to say NO when necessary, your
    courage to say I come first this time, I matter, I am
    beautiful, I am valuable, I am good enough and I
    deserve excellent care (especially from myself).
    By beginning to identify these emotions you will
already begin the process of healing. Learning to meditate
(see Chapter 5) may assist you in releasing some of the

damaging emotions, but with longstanding issues that may point to depression or anxiety, it is advisable you set aside some time for a few sessions of counselling, either with a psychologist or through an (EAP) employee assistant wellness programme at your work.

The cardiac check this week also requires you to check the entire circle of your life. Just as your heart is the centre of your body, so you are at the centre of all your roles: you as a mother, in the workplace, as partner, in a community. The concept of an embrace is indeed a circle. Each part of you is part of this circle, just like the slices of a pie. Take a look at these seven areas (shown below). Is any one area neglected? Or is one area receiving almost all your energy and time to the detriment of other aspects of your life?

Do you have a balance? Balance does not mean perfectly in alignment. It means a dynamic flow between outwards and inwards, between busy and restful, between giving and taking, between all the various aspects that make up you in your world. Some areas do demand much more than others.

This is *your* Action Plan. You need to step out of all your roles for a moment and prioritise.

Balance is not a point at which you arrive. It is continually moving and shifting. You are the driver and director of your time and your energy.

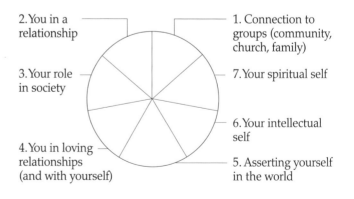

2. You in a relationship

3. Your role in society

4. You in loving relationships (and with yourself)

1. Connection to groups (community, church, family)

7. Your spiritual self

6. Your intellectual self

5. Asserting yourself in the world

🌿
Week 2: Nurturing the nurturer
🌿

This is the week to begin to nurture yourself and implement your self-pampering strategy. Perhaps start taking care of yourself in a new way. It is beginning to treat yourself with compassion and attentive care. Taking care of your body includes a good sleep routine, an excellent nutrition programme and dynamic exercise. Those components of your personal action plan follow on from here and are designed for Months Three, Four and Five. You can choose to implement them together with your 'embracing' month. But the reason for this coming first is that up until now, nurturing has probably been last on your personal agenda (if at all!).

Below are a few suggestions for you to begin a self-pampering plan. Indulge in one or all of these suggestions this week, and remember to continue throughout this month and incorporate it into your schedule.

Flowers

Do not wait for someone else to buy you flowers. Buy a beautiful bunch especially for yourself today! Choose fresh flowers that appeal to your senses. Do not choose something that looks good in your entrance hall or living room. Choose what *you* love and place them next to your bed. Each day notice their beauty and scent and nurture your soul with a small measure of this beauty.

Candles

Candles somehow represent an atmosphere of hope and light and joy. A candle provides a sensory experience with its flickering flame and exotic aroma. It also provides an ethereal quality that perhaps represents a spiritual element. Light a candle or a few candles at the end of a long day, allowing the gentle light and aroma to enliven your senses. You could do this in your bathroom while you pamper yourself or even in your bedroom or on the dinner table.

Bath

Very little can match the soothing, therapeutic effects of a long soak in a fragrant bathtub. You can easily enhance this experience and use the following to sooth all your senses:
+ smell – exquisite aromatherapy oils or candles
+ touch – moisturising luxurious soaps and creams
+ hearing – relaxing mood music
+ sight – dim lights and flickering flames
+ taste – fragrant herb tea or even better an indulgent steaming hot chocolate.

Treat

Treats are not just for kids. A treat is SOMETHING special for SOMEONE special. Treat yourself sometimes. It does not have to be expensive to feel valuable. A deep sleep one afternoon on the weekend is a real luxurious treat. A walk in a botanical garden may be what enlivens you. It may be any of the 'time outs' or pamperings in next week's programme. Or it may be stopping for ten minutes at a coffee shop in the middle of your day for steaming, sweet, creamy cappuccino. A treat may be buying yourself something you really want such as a new music CD or recipe book.

Week 3
Take good care

Only you can identify what you really need in order to take excellent care. Do you want a session of pampering, do you need some mental stimulation or perhaps an activity to feed your soul? Possibly all you really need is a comfortable bed and a catch-up on sleep. You ought to make an effort to block off time each week for at least one of these four aspects of your personal action plan:
+ Extra rest
+ Pampering
+ Time-outs
+ Recreation

You obviously cannot manage all this week or all four aspects every week. Make a commitment for at least one session per week to continue to nurture the nurturer. Interchange these activities. This week you devote your time to extra rest, the week thereafter may be a pedicure and the following week is a trip to the nursery to buy some seedlings for your garden. Make sure you sit for a while in the nursery tea garden and savour a cappuccino before you leave.

You may find you have time for more than one nurturing session – you can fit in a massage on a Tuesday evening and a sleep on a Saturday afternoon or you're able to set aside a half-hour for browsing through the bookstore one day and still manage a lecture one evening.

🌿
Week 4: Nurture your beauty, nurture your sexuality
🌿

Become aware of what you can do to enhance your beauty and your sexuality and step up your life. This week requires you to be extremely honest with yourself. Sure, you need to be realistic and reach a level of self-acceptance, but know that there is much that can be done to look after your beauty and your skin throughout your life.

Beauty tips

✦ Every woman has some aspect of beauty – nurture yours!

✦ A healthy balanced diet with lots of fresh fruits and vegetables is essential for a great skin (see Health Action Plan in Chapter 3).

✦ Keep well hydrated: seven to eight glasses of water a day.

✦ Sleep is vital: seven to eight hours of sleep a night.

✦ Exercise, especially in fresh air (with sunscreen).

✦ Daily beauty regime: cleanser, toner and moisturiser. It need not be expensive, but should match your skin type and age.

✦ Use sun protection daily throughout summer and winter. Sun damage is the major contributor to skin damage and ageing.

✦ Remember that beauty is so much more! It is a depth of character, expression of your real self, a unique personality, compassion and caring, inherently a deep part of you.

To nurture your sexual energy requires an honest appraisal. Tips to nurture your sexuality (this week and every week!):
✦ Begin to apply the principles of nurturing:
  ☆ self-acceptance
  ☆ self-love
  ☆ identify your needs.
✦ It is essential that you become vigilant about *safe sex*.
✦ Know that good sex demands communication, relationship building, and a willingness to express your vulnerability.
✦ Begin to 'let go'. This one area of your life that does not need tight control!
✦ If there are relationship issues, consider a few sessions of combined counselling. If you both care for each other, with a little insight and perspective you can achieve real closeness.
✦ Prepare for sex. Think about it, fantasise. Identify what it is you would like. Pamper yourself . Use candles and a relaxing soak in the tub.
✦ You can become the driver! Initiate and ask for what you need. Remember all the health benefits too!

CHAPTER 3

Eat

Introduction

Eating impacts on every area of your life, and is the centre of many social and cultural occasions. Food is nutrition but it also provides pleasure and comfort. Food provides sustenance and energy but it is about connections, communication and memories, too. If you are part of a family, you will be involved in endless shopping, preparation and cooking of meals. You will be concerned about finicky eaters, packing nutritious lunch boxes and trying to keep the family healthy.

Your own relationship with food may be one of huge pleasure and enjoyment or it may involve guilt and remorse. Unfortunately, for many women food has become an enemy. In the pursuit and maintenance of a good physique, so much food has become forbidden, but no food really needs to be prohibited. Eating is an area over which you have so much control. You need to make really good choices about the best quality nutrition and allow yourself to partake of the physical and emotional pleasures of eating.

Nutrition Quick Quiz: How much do you know?

1. What packs more nutrients?
   ☆ red pepper ....
   ☆ green pepper ....

2. Which is better for you: a chicken breast or a drumstick?
   ☆ white meat ....
   ☆ brown meat ....

3. Carrots belong to the same family as:
   ☆ potatoes ....
   ☆ radishes ....
   ☆ parsley ....
   ☆ peanuts ....

(Nutrition Quick Quiz: *Continued overleaf*)

4. If you are going to drink alcohol which is the most nutritious?
   ☆ dark beer ....
   ☆ golden beer ....
   ☆ spirits ....
   ☆ red wine ....

5. Which is more nutritious?
   ☆ peanut butter ....
   ☆ strawberry jam ....

6. Could chocolate possibly be good for you and which one should you choose?
   ☆ milk chocolate ....
   ☆ dark chocolate ....
   ☆ white chocolate ....

Answers

ANSWER 1
A red pepper 10 points
A green pepper 0 points
A red pepper has more vitamins and nutrients. The level of carotene, an important antioxidant, is nine times higher in a red pepper. And the red kind has twice the vitamin C of the green.

ANSWER 2
Dark meat chicken 10 points
White meat chicken 0 points
Surprise! The dark meat contains a special protein called myoglobin, which is full of iron. And it also has more than twice the amount of zinc as the white meat.

So, although the drumstick has more fat than the breast, it also has more nutrients.

ANSWER 3
Potatoes 0
Radishes 0
Parsley10
Peanuts 0
Parsley is the right answer. Carrots are high in beta- and alpha-carotene. Not only are carrots powerful antioxidants, but the beta-carotene helps metabolise vitamin A in the body and improve night vision.

ANSWER 4:
Dark beer 5
Golden beer 0
Spirits 0
Red wine 5
Dark beer has more phytochemicals (see table on page 115) from the grain used to make it than there are in a lighter beer. Phytochemicals help keep blood from clotting. Red wine contains phenols which act as antioxidants i.e. neutralising damaged cells. It also contains resveretrol which has shown in preliminary studies to have anti-ageing properties.

ANSWER 5
Peanut butter 10
Strawberry jam 0
Peanut butter – chunky or creamy – has 190 calories per two-tablespoon serving. And, although it's high in fat, the fat is mostly the mono-unsaturated kind. So choose whichever type you prefer and enjoy (unless you are overweight and on a markedly restricted calorie diet)!

ANSWER 6
Milk chocolate 0
Dark chocolate 10
White chocolate 0
The truth is that dark chocolate is actually good for you, especially in preventing heart disease. Chocolate contains the phenols that are in red wine. Chocolate has also recently been shown to contain epicatechin, an antioxidant from the group of phytochemicals called flavonoids, which may reduce blood clots and decrease clogged arteries. Dark chocolate has more cocoa-bean extract, so it has a higher phenol count than milk chocolate. White chocolate has no phenols at all because it's not made from cocoa beans. While a little dark choc is good, a lot is not better. Chocolate is still loaded with calories, so you will have to cut back on something else. Remember to eat the best quality dark chocolate which has the highest concentration of cocoa.

Scoring
0-20 = You are a nutrition novice
You need to arm yourself with plenty of up-to-date nutrition information! Read right through the chapter and you will be amazed at what the new responsible research has demonstrated.

30-40 = You are a food enthusiast
You are well on your way to establishing healthy eating habits. Now that you know what kind of chocolate you should eat, read on to find out what carbs, proteins, fats, fruits and veggies you should be consuming each day.

50-70 = You are a foodie expert
You can rattle off the latest cutting edge nutrition stories at any dinner party. You know the nutrient value of sprouts, sushi and carrot cake. Keep going but make sure you are up to the moment with food news, so read on . . .

Katherine's story
I'm sure you know at least one remarkable story where someone went on a new diet and her cancer went into remission or her arthritis disappeared. You have also heard that right now the very best weight loss programme will guarantee results like no other! Every day there are miracle stories attributed to a nutritional programme. I am not a cynic. I do believe that healing is always possible. And astonishing recoveries do take place far too often to dismiss as random or coincidental.

The power of sound nutrition is indeed huge. What you eat will have an impact on all areas of your health. But all illness and poor health does not stem solely from poor nutrition, and changing your diet alone (regardless of how restrictive) will not be enough to bring about healing unless it is part of a total health plan.

In 1994 Katherine (39), a successful professional, was diagnosed with hypertension. She had just given birth to her first child after a healthy pregnancy. It seemed that the high blood pressure was transient and would settle after a few weeks. After weekly checks her blood pressure seemed to be consistently high and so she was started on anti-hypertensives. She gained over 20 kilograms with the pregnancy which was difficult to lose. She was experiencing problems in her marriage and became clinically depressed, and was unresponsive to supportive psychotherapy; eventually she needed medication. Smoking, eating, frustrated and depressed, she was on a downward spiral.

Katherine was fairly unmotivated to begin a healthy action programme. However, while feeding her baby one day, she suddenly experienced a loss of vision and paralysis which looked just like a stroke. She was rushed to hospital and immediately admitted. The episode thankfully subsided after 24 hours and was reclassified as a TIA (Transient Ischaemic Attack).

It unfortunately often requires a scare to jolt us into action. Katherine began a responsible weight reduction programme. After three months she had shed 20 kilograms and was not only in great shape, exercising and feeling good, she was also able to reduce and finally stop her blood pressure medication. Her blood pressure has remained completely normal over the past 10 years. She has managed to turn her life and health around, and reverse her high risk for heart disease and stroke.

My story
I love food! I enjoy meals prepared with care, love and passion. I generally prefer healthy foodstuffs but have a weakness for the indulgences, too.

I suppose you would not look at me and think *'there goes a fat woman'* but I am by no means at a perfect or ideal weight and size. There are times when I am completely at peace with myself, my voluptuous curves or plain 'doughy' (as my children call it) areas of flesh. I feel great about myself, knowing that this less than perfect body has served me well, has carried my many children, feels strong and fit, is at a healthy Body Mass Index (BMI) (see page 311) and generally looks good in decent clothes. Most importantly, I feel healthy. There are other times when I decide to check out my body fat, or get on the scale, or the clothes feel a little tight, that I feel that terrible self-loathing creeping in. I am tempted to try yet again to shed a few kilos or get my body fat level down a little.

I have tried and tested all the diets. In my youth I chose a vegetarian path for 10 years, and then progressed through all the fads. Way back in the 1980s Scarsdale, Mayo Clinic and Weight Watchers were the rage. The last two decades encouraged me to try out food combining, the Blood Group Diet, the Zone Diet and finally Atkins and South Beach – all of which I have commented on later in this chapter (pages 121-126). All these eating programmes took place against the backdrop of a journey of spiritual, emotional and personal growth. My focus was to attempt to integrate my body consciousness with all the other facets of who I am.

It took a serious bout of illness and many months of intense fatigue and nausea to get me to do the fashionable 'detox'. I cut out wheat, dairy, meat and anything processed and preserved. So I basically ate brown rice and avocados with a bit of fruit for a few months. My recovery was slow but complete and was due to much more than a detox diet.

With the passage of time, maturity, self-acceptance and common sense, I attempt to live by the principles outlined in the SELF diet. Good nutrition is powerful fuel for your body. But deprivation is harmful. I use the 80-20 rule: 80 per cent of the food I eat is best quality, most nourishing fresh foodstuffs (plenty of fresh vegetables, fruit, grains, good oils, fish) and 20 per cent allows for some less than perfect food – occasional smoked foods, preserved foods and delicious treats.

What exactly is 'A Healthy Diet'?

A healthy diet is certainly the cornerstone of a healthy lifestyle. But it is hard to know exactly what a healthy diet is. As with many things, there are fashions and fads with food, but what is fact and what is fiction? The bookstore shelves are overflowing with diet and nutrition books, and the more you read, the more confused you get!

I do not want to add to your confusion but rather want to outline some simple and clear principles to promote better health. Of course, there is huge health value in following a nutritious diet plan, and it is now established that certain dietary practices cause as well as prevent a wide range of diseases. In many instances, changing your diet *can* alter the pattern of your illness and facilitate healing and wellbeing. Your body has an innate capacity for repair and healing, and good nutrition can stimulate and enhance these pathways.

But do not believe anyone who tells you that it is all about what you eat. There are two important myths that need to be dismissed: firstly that all illness is from poor nutrition, and secondly that the right diet can cure anything. You are a multifaceted being and all aspects (your mental, emotional and spiritual life) will affect you health and healing.

Looking back over the past 20 years of food trends, we have seen in the 1980s the carbohydrate craze and the complete cutting out of fat. Then came the 1990s where fat was no longer so bad, as long as you were having the good fats. And in the first few years of this millennium, it has been protein that has been highlighted as the hero, especially for weight loss. There certainly is some value in all three decades of nutrition wisdom, but also much erroneous thinking. Even the FDA's (United States Food and Drug Administration) Food Pyramid, which was seen as a gold standard of nutrition, has been drastically adapted (see page 145).

No single approach has ownership of good health. There is no quick fix to weight loss and optimal health. You will do well by implementing the following 10 principles into your life which are all based on good science and preventive health. These are not my fads or fashions but rather a structure designed to empower you as a woman to take charge of your own health and the health of your family.

10 Healthy Diet Principles
1. Quality Counts
Eat the best quality foods you can afford: good quality proteins (e.g. salmon), good quality carbs (e.g. heavy grainy breads), good quality fats (olive oil and avocados).

2. Fabulously Fresh
When possible eat it fresh! This will reduce the intake of additives, preservatives and colourants.

3. Preferably Plant
Increase the plant-based part of your diet: plenty of fresh vegetables, salad and fruit.

95

Eat at least three fruit servings and four to five vegetable/salad servings per day (more if you like).The South African Cancer Association recommends seven to nine portions per day.

Include varieties with strong antioxidants which help repair the body, e.g. broccoli, spinach, sweet potato, beetroot (see Table 4 on page 108).

4. Minimise Meat
Cut down red meat intake (enjoy occasionally).

5. Fish Feast
Replace some of your family's meat meals with fish such as salmon, sardines and fatty fish – they contain wonderful omega fats which are so healthy. Non-fatty fish is an extremely good source of protein.

6. Full of Fibre
Increase your intake of fibre in the form of pulses, legumes and nuts.

7. Reduce Refined
Cut down refined sugar, refined white flour, biscuits, cakes, etc. *This does not mean eliminate them! You can still enjoy in moderation!*

8. Foolish Fats
Avoid and cut down on 'bad' fats (saturated and toxic fats or transfatty acids). Saturated fats are found in fatty cuts of red meat, full-cream dairy products, deep-fried pies and pastries. But enjoy 'good' fats (monosaturated fats)! Olive oil, if cold pressed and virgin, is great for health, as is canola oil and the fat within avocados.

9. Hydrated Health
Drink fresh water (preferably filtered) and energising herbal teas. Moderate caffeine intake.

10. Soul celebration
Enjoy your food!

Best Nutrition Principles

The squabbles continue through the media, in books and even with the experts. *'Isn't too much protein bad for you?''No, high protein will assist with weight loss!''I thought fats make you fat?''What is all the new talk about carbs and starch making you fat?'*

With so much discussion and debate over which diet is best and more importantly which of the food groups are to blame for obesity and poor health, the most important factor has been overlooked. **Eat the best quality foodstuffs in each of the food groups.** Excess of any of the components (including protein) will lead to poor health and weight gain. There are only two words you need to incorporate into your new eating plan: QUALITY and MODERATION.

Intake of all the food groups is essential for optimum health, but there are good and bad choices. Ask yourself these two important questions when deciding what to eat:

1. What is damaging to my body which I should eliminate or reduce?
2. What is valuable and energising that I should include or increase in my diet?

Best fats

When you think of the word fat, you think of that deposit of doughy rolls across your abdomen and hips and the bumps of cellulite around your thighs. This is just the excess deposit of fat in tissue called adipose tissue.

Fats and oils are essential to your health. They are the components of vital internal tissues, organs and cells. Brain function, nerve transmission, cell membranes and production of hormones and enzymes all require essential fatty acids. Fats are a source of energy supply for the body, too.

Many good fats must be consumed in your diet. Obviously, if you are overweight and need to lose kilograms and body fat, you must reduce your total fat intake. But the blanket approach to 'zero fat' tolerance is an unhealthy concept.

Research has linked a diet high in saturated fats to numerous cancers, heart disease and strokes, but the good fats have a cardioprotective effect and nourish the cells of your body.

The three basic groupings of dietary fat are: *saturated fats*, and unsaturated fats which are grouped into *polyunsaturated* and *mono-unsaturated fats*.

1. *Saturated fats* (SFAs) are the harmful, damaging fat substances found in animal fats, butter fat, coconut, palm and palm kernel oil. Cut down on your intake of saturated fats. If you have a cholesterol or lipid problem, cut them out altogether as they aggravate cholesterol accumulation. Saturated fats are abundant in meats, especially pork and lamb, but also beef and in poultry skin, as well as full-cream dairy produce and butter. You may be unaware that there are also vegetable saturated fats. Coconut, palm and palm kernel oils are often hidden in many products, such as in biscuits, cereals and even 'healthy' muesli. The easiest way to cut down is to eat fewer animal products and processed baked goods, and more fresh fruit and vegetables.

2. *Polyunsaturated fats*, also called PUFAs (polyunsaturated fatty acids), are found in sunflower, corn, flaxseed, soybean, walnut and sesame oil. These unsaturated oils in their natural state are generally good for you. They are the conventional cooking or salad oils that you buy in the supermarket, but are not as beneficial as the mono-unsaturated fats (see below). They are best used cold as to deep-fry food in these oils can turn them to saturated fats.

   Unfortunately in their processing many of them undergo chemical reactions rendering them harmful. Margarine in particular is affected. The good sunflower and other PUFA oils are made toxic by the formation of what is called 'trans-fatty acids'. These trans-fatty acids have been shown to increase fatty deposits in blood vessels as well as cause cellular damage, resulting in many degenerative disorders.

3. *Mono-unsaturated fats* (MUFAs) are the outstanding choice for your health. They are found in avocado and olive oil as well as macadamia nuts. These are the fats that you should be eating. Avocados are extremely nutritious, containing an excellent source of oil. Even if you have a half or quarter per day, try to include avos in your diet. They are wonderful for your skin, too.

Olive oil is the one outstanding fat and should be part of your diet even if you are on a weight loss programme. It must be cold pressed and virgin or extra virgin because when heat-treated it becomes damaged. Some commercially available products add cheaper oils to the olive oil. Watch out for this. Olive oil is a really expensive choice but use it sparingly. If you cannot afford it, eat more avocados.

Canola oil in its pure form is a mono-unsaturated fat but during processing undergoes some chemical and heat damage.

Two very important fats that you should include in your diet are the omega-6 and omega-3 fatty acids. [Note: You generally get more than enough omega-6 in your diet; the importance is the balance and ratio of omega-6 and omega-3.] They are essential for your hormone balance throughout life, and have a protective effect on your heart and blood vessels. They also are excellent for your cellular function, joints, bones and mental function. Omega 3-fatty acids are found in fish, especially salmon and mackerel, and in walnuts. If you are not eating enough fresh fish, it is advised that you take an omega fatty acid supplement.

Best proteins
Protein is the buzz word in many current diets, including Dr Atkins, the Zone and the South Beach diets. As carbohydrates have unfortunately been downgraded as a good nutritional source, protein somehow has taken centre stage. Certainly proteins are essential dietary requirements but an excess of protein may be harmful and damaging.

Your remarkable body is constantly regenerating and repairing damaged cells and renewing all tissues. Cells die all the time and new cells are laid down in all structures of your body. For example, every 28 days your entire skin is shed and new skin cells laid down. For this it needs building blocks in the form of proteins which are composed of amino acids.

As a woman you need to eat a moderate amount of protein each day, once or twice a day is generally more than adequate. Children certainly need protein for growth but women require extra protein only during pregnancy, if convalescing from an illness and if exercising and training really hard. Choose to eat a nice portion of protein at one or two meals a day or a small portion with each meal.

Much of the data regarding weight loss or maintenance of your ideal body weight is focused on metabolism of glucose and the role of insulin. Ideally you would like the glucose and fuel to be absorbed as slowly as possible into your bloodstream so as not to stimulate a huge insulin surge (see Carbohydrates below). As the carbohydrate content of your meal is broken down into glucose, which is quickly absorbed into your bloodstream, protein is a most effective substrate in slowing down the absorption of the glucose.

The RDA (Recommended Daily Allowance) for protein is age and gender dependent. Assuming you are an adult female older than 25 years, you would need 50 grams of protein per day. This is equivalent to one chicken breast, or two eggs, or a small piece of meat (the size of your palm), or half a cup of cooked butter beans. This is all you need for the entire day! So although you do not need to eat it with every meal, there is value in adding a small amount of protein to each meal along with your vegetables, salads and carbohydrates. The rationale for this stems from the concept of slowing down the entry of fuel (primarily glucose) into your bloodstream.

There is no nutritional value in eating more than the protein RDA if your body doesn't need it. Protein cannot be stored in the body and any excess protein is excreted. Furthermore, excessive daily protein intake (over 2g per kilo, per day) can overload the kidneys. High levels of protein in your diet are also associated with increased loss of calcium, which may be harmful for bones and increase the risk of osteoporosis in later life. An excessive intake of protein may also be responsible for some allergies, degenerative conditions and immune sensitivities.

Types of protein
Animal proteins are red meat in the form of beef, lamb and pork; white meat in the form of poultry; dairy products, cheeses and all types of fish. Plant proteins include legumes and pulses i.e. beans, lentils, chickpeas and soya products.

100

A tremendous amount of information shows that a predominantly animal-based diet is a major factor in the development of heart disease, cancer, strokes, arthritis and many other degenerative diseases. It is now the recommendation of many health and medical organisations that your diet should focus primarily on plant-based foods. Such a diet is thought to offer protection against development of chronic degenerative illness.

There are many advantages of eating more vegetable sources of protein. Animal protein contains high saturated fats, an extremely concentrated protein load to your kidneys, as well as unnecessary hormones that are harmful. Some poultry and meat products contain injected female hormones (oestrogen). Although there are no conclusive scientific studies, it is speculated that this may be one of the contributing factors to the very early development of puberty in young girls and the increased incidence of female cancers. I am not advocating your becoming a vegetarian. By eating red meat occasionally and chicken once or twice a week you will probably be doing almost no harm, but a chicken meal four nights a week, and red meat the other three is certainly not in your best health interests.

Vegetable protein, such as soya, in addition to its nourishing properties, absorbs excess circulating oestrogen hormones which may play a role in preventing breast and prostatic cancers. The Japanese population, perhaps due to their high intake of soya, have an insignificant incidence of breast and prostate cancer. This is a controversial area of nutritional research. In addition, processed soya products are often criticised for their high fat and preservative content. They are not perfect foodstuffs but are valuable sources of good plant protein and fibre, and to use them as a substitute for a meat meal is certainly recommended. Soya products are also a much healthier option to feed your family instead of processed meat, sausages and burgers.

Fish: Increasing the quantity of fish in your diet is essential. This is an excellent source of low-fat protein as well as omega-3 fatty acids which are found abundantly in salmon, mackerel, herring and sardines. Omega-

3 fatty acids are vital to your health as they improve your mental function and cellular repair, and show marked anti-inflammatory and healthy heart properties.

Dairy: Unless you have a specific allergy, dairy is a wonderful source of calcium and protein for women. I recommend the low-fat varieties as full-cream dairy is a saturated fat source. Although there is some debate about the presence of a growth hormone within milk that may be linked in some way to breast cancer, there is at present no conclusive evidence, but perhaps if you have a very strong family history of breast cancer, cut down on your dairy.

Best carbohydrates
Whether you are at your ideal weight, three kilos or thirty kilos over-weight or underweight, you need a nutritious diet rich in vitamins, minerals and fibre. Good carbohydrates, like vegetables, fruit, wholegrain cereals, oats, beans, soya, potatoes, wholewheat bread, pasta and rice, provide good nutrition. Vegetables, in particular, contain a range of phytochemicals, enzymes and other micronutrients that are essential for an efficient metabolism and a healthy diet.

Carbohydrates, essentially starches and sugar, supply energy and play a role in the functioning of the entire body, including the brain. Excessive intake of carbs will certainly be stored as fat but adequate or moderate intake will be used as an efficient source of fuel. Carbs are readily usable by the body and are clean-burning fuels. Your body adapts to a wide range of different carbohydrates. Starch itself in moderation is a great foodstuff but the indiscriminate intake of masses of starch or sugar will certainly lead to weight gain.

While thousands of women (and men) say they've reduced their weight through carb-reduction, nutrition experts remain divided over these diets. Critics contend that dieters who have lost weight did so because they trimmed calories, not cut carbs. On this point, studies are mixed.

But both the low-carb and high-carb advocates agree that it's best to get any carbohydrates from high-fibre, whole-food sources, often referred to as complex or low Glycaemic Index carbs. Wholegrain bread, wholegrain pasta and brown rice, for instance, are favoured over white bread, white-flour pasta and white rice. Refined (white) sugar, high in both calories and carbs but lacking nutrients, is discouraged by both camps.

Glycaemic Index

The key issue in carb consumption is the Glycaemic Index (GI) – a measure of the effect of foods on blood sugars. Studies have shown that wholegrains and other foods with low GIs can help keep your blood sugar levels stable and maintain a feeling of fullness. The low GI carbs may therefore restrain hunger and in this way, help you lose weight. Heavier, grainier high-fibre starch (low GI) is healthier for digestion. Low GI foods, such as sweet potatoes, brown rice, dense breads and pasta cooked *al dente* provide energy in a slow and sustained release form, facilitating the smooth use of calories and alleviating hunger for longer periods. High GI foods, such as potatoes, white short-grain rice and refined bread, provide bursts of energy that may be followed by hunger and general depletion. This does not mean that you should now eliminate all high GI foods, but that the proportion of low GI foods in your diet should be greater. (See also page 116, Insulin and carbohydrates.)

Finding the GI spot!

Foods only appear on the GI index if they contain a carbohydrate. This explains why you won't find foods like fresh meat, chicken, fish, eggs and cheese in GI lists. However, you may find some processed foods like sausages or chicken nuggets in a GI list because they contain flour.

Low Glycaemic Index foods (55 or less)

Include some of these foods in each meal or snack, but go for low-fat choices where possible, such as skimmed milk. To lose weight, watch your portion sizes, stick to small servings. These foods are not all non-fattening foods. Peanuts, crisps and chocolate should be minimised or eliminated on a calorie-controlled weight reduction plan. They move slowly into the bloodstream, but in this case because of their higher fat content.

Medium Glycaemic Index foods (56 to 69)

You may include a few of these foods each day, but again, limit portion sizes if you want to lose weight.

High Glycaemic Index foods (70 or more)

Swap these foods for those with a low GI value or eat them together with a low GI food. Eating a potato with its skin on, together with baked beans, for example, will lower the GI value of that whole meal.

Best fibre

Dietary fibre, or 'roughage', is not a nutrient but is nevertheless an important component of your diet. The fact that it passes through your body without being absorbed is the main reason why fibre is vital.

What is fibre?

Dietary fibre is the undigested remains of plant materials. It is found only in foods derived from plants, and all plant food provides some fibre; how much depends on whether it has been processed or not. Unpeeled fruit and vegetables and wholemeal or wholegrain cereal foods will provide the most. For example, brown rice contains seven times more fibre than white rice because it still contains the outer layers of the grain. The various components of dietary fibre found in different foods are called cellulose, hemicellulose, pectin and lignin.

Dietary fibre can be soluble or insoluble. *Soluble fibre* dissolves in your gut to form a kind of gel. This slows down the release of glucose into your bloodstream. It is therefore good for diabetics. It can also reduce your risk of heart disease by reducing your blood cholesterol levels. Soluble fibre is present in fruit, vegetables, pulses (e.g. baked beans, lentils) and foods containing oats, barley or rye.

Insoluble fibre, on the other hand, has a sponge-like effect in your gut, soaking up water and swelling in size. This effect produces a feeling of fullness and adds bulk to the gut contents, making waste matter heavier and speeding it through the large intestine. It is therefore thought to

Table 1: Low GI Foods

Food	GI	Food	GI
★ Roasted and salted peanuts	14	Peaches	42
Low-fat plain yoghurt with sweetener	14	Porridge (e.g. oats or mielie meal)	42
Cherries (fresh), berries	22	Lentil soup	44
Grapefruit	25	Oranges	44
Barley	25	Macaroni	45
Lentils	26	Grapes (green and black)	46
Full-cream milk	27	Peas (fresh and frozen)	48
Dried apricots	31	Baked beans in tomato sauce	48
Butter beans	31	Carrots, boiled	49
Fettucine pasta	32	★ Dark chocolate	49
Skimmed milk	32	Kiwi fruit	52
Low-fat fruit yoghurt	33	Wholemeal bread	53
Wholewheat spaghetti	37	★ Crisps	54
Apples	38	Specially formulated low GI breakfast cereals	54
Pears	38	Banana	55
Noodles (cooked *al dente*)	40	Raw oatbran	55
Spaghetti (cooked *al dente*)	41	Sweetcorn (fresh corn on cob and tinned, plain)	55
All Bran flakes (depending on brand)	42		
Chickpeas, canned	42		

★ Because they have a low GI does not mean they are healthy

reduce the risk of constipation and possibly even cancers of the digestive system. Cereal and grain products (rice, pasta, barley, rye), especially wholemeal varieties, and fibrous vegetables (e.g. carrots and celery) are primary sources of insoluble fibre.

Table 2: Moderate GI Foods

Food	GI	Food	GI
Muesli, non-toasted	56	Raisins	64
Boiled potatoes (big)	56	Shortbread biscuit	64
Sultanas	56	Couscous	65
Pita bread	57	Rye bread	65
Basmati rice	58	Pineapple, fresh	66
Honey	58	Sweet melon	67
Digestive biscuit	59	Croissant	67
Ice cream	61	Rye crispbread	69
New potatoes	62	Weetbix	69
Apricots, canned in syrup	64	Brown bread	69

Table 3: High GI Foods

Food	GI	Food	GI
Mashed potato	70	Jelly beans	80
White bread	70	Rice cakes	82
Watermelon	72	Rice popped cereal	82
Bagel	72	Cornflakes	84
Bran breakfast flakes	74	Potato with skin	85
French fries	75	Baguette	95
Coco Pops	77	White rice, steamed	98

Fibre is good for you. Unlike sugar, salt and fat, fibre is something you could eat more of. A most important thing to remember is that fibre in an isolated form, such as bran (the outer layers of cereal grain), is not the answer because bran can actually reduce the absorption of minerals. Fibre is far more beneficial if it is consumed as an integral part of food, rather than as bran supplements or fibre-containing drinks.

Best plant foods (fruit and vegetables)

Eating fresh fruit and vegetables in abundance is the cornerstone of good nutrition. It boosts your natural energy and protects and heals your body. The National Cancer Association recommends five to nine servings of fruit and vegetables every day. This should be a combination of fresh raw vegetables in salads, cooked green, yellow and orange vegetables as well as three or four fruit serves, depending on your particular diet.

Superfoods – Phytochemicals

The latest buzzword in nutrition is phytochemicals (pronounced 'fight-o-chemicals', they fight to protect your health). These chemicals are found in fruit and vegetables. They augment immunity and reduce the risk of cancer and other serious illnesses. The cells of your body are continually exposed to oxidation damage through pollution, sunlight, stress, smoke, chemicals and environmental toxins. Phytochemicals have an anti-oxidant effect on cells which mop up and neutralise the damage.

They seem to work together with other compounds rather than each on their own. They may help slow the ageing process and reduce your risk of many diseases, including stroke, heart disease, cancer and osteoporosis. They have many fancy biochemical names such as:

+ **Caretonoids** are the pigment responsible for the colour of many red, green, yellow and orange fruit and vegetables. They are a large family of phytochemicals which include *alpha-carotene, beta-carotene, lutein, lycopene, cryptoxanthin and zeaxanthin.* They protect the body by decreasing the risk of heart disease, stroke, blindness and certain cancers. They may also help slow the ageing process, improve lung function and reduce diabetes complications

   Beta-carotene: Found in squash, pumpkins, carrots, sweet potatoes, butternut, mangoes, apricots, papaya, kiwi fruit

   Lutein: Found in broccoli, spinach and greens

   Lycopene: Found in tomatoes, red peppers, watermelon

   Zeaxanthin: Found in squash, corn and spinach

+ **Polyphenols and flavonoids:** Found in celery, cranberries, apples, cherries, tea, red wine, parsley, eggplant and tomatoes. And even in

107

Table 4: Nutrients in fruit and vegetables

Fruit/Vegetable	Vitamins and nutrients	Phytochemicals and antioxidant
Apples	Vitamin C and pectin	Polyphenols and flavonoids
Avocados	Vitamin C, vitamin E, potassium, mono-unsaturated fat (= good oil)	
Bananas	Great source of potassium. High levels of vitamin B6	
Broccoli	Vitamin C, vitamin A and calcium, selenium and fibre	Huge amount of antioxidants, beta-carotene
Carrots	Vitamin A	Very high in beta-carotene
Celery	High in calcium	Polyphenols and flavonoids
Cranberries	High in vitamin C and vitamin A	Protective phytochemical in red and purple fruit (anthocyanins)
Garlic		Allicin
Grapes	High in vitamin C	Red grapes high in phytochemical is anthocyanins (as in all red and purple fruit)
Grapefruit	High in vitamin C and fibre	Monoterpines
Green leafy vegetables: kale, cabbage, sprouts, watercress	Vitamin C, vitamin A and calcium	Huge amount of antioxidants, isothocyanates and lutein, beta-carotene
Onions		Organosulfur compounds
Oranges	Prime source of vitamin C	Monoterpines
Peppers	Vitamin C and high iron and potassium	Beta-carotene, capsaicin
Pineapples	Contains enzymes and rich in vitamin C	
Potatoes	Great source of fibre and vitamin C	Saponins mop up damaged cells
Spinach	Rich in iron and chlorophyll, vitamins C and E	Isothocyanates and lutein
Tomatoes		Lycopene and other antioxidants

General

'Keeps the doctor away'. Keeps cholesterol in check and binds to heavy metals, clearing them out of your system. Is a low GI carbohydrate.

Super for women and anti-ageing as they encourage collagen production in the skin (soft, supple, youthful looking skin). Excellent nutrition.

Good for the nervous system, helps with fatigue and depression and muscle and leg cramps. Good before bed as aids in the release of sleep-inducing agents.

Perhaps the most useful antioxidant food you can eat.
Great for building strong bones.

Best eaten fresh. It is possible to overdose, especially on carrot juice – you can turn orange!

Acts as a natural diuretic.

Protects against urinary tract infections because of antibacterial properties. May have anti-cancer properties.

Contains allicin which acts as a natural antibiotic and lowers blood pressure. Thought to protect against cancer and heart disease by lowering cholesterol. May improve memory.

Prevents gum infections.

May reduce cholesterol.

Powerful antioxidant foods, as is broccoli. Great for building strong bones.

Shown to raise the good cholesterol HDL and perhaps reduce stroke risk and anti-cancer properties.

Thought to aid immune system.

Enzymes may aid digestion.

Sweet potatoes are the queen of vegetable kingdom with their higher nutrients. Do not eat green, black or sprouted spuds.

Excellent for warding off fatigue and anaemia and possibly cancer. According to British Medical Journal, spinach is the most effective vegetable in preventing cataracts.

Wonder food full of lycopene, cooked tomatoes work best, even processed tomato sauce is outstanding.

dark chocolate! [Note: Polyphenols and flavonoids keep cholesterol from gathering in blood vessels, they reduce the risk of blood clots and slow down the clogging of arteries.]

✦ **Isoflavones:** Commonly known as phytooestrogens, they have actions similar to the hormone oestrogen. They act as antioxidants and tumor suppressors, and may improve cholesterol, prevent bone loss and suppress enzymes. They are mainly found in soya products and some seeds.

✦ **Isothiocyanates** are found in cauliflower, broccoli, turnips, kohlrabi, cabbage and greens. They are thought to block the steroid hormones that promote breast and prostate cancers.

✦ **Monoterpines:** They block proteins that stimulate cell growth and cancer formation. They are found in citrus fruits, especially in the peels.

✦ **Organosulfur compounds** come from the allium family and are found in garlic, leeks, onions, chives. They may have benefits for the immune system, reduce cholesterol and render harmful cancer-producing substances harmless.

✦ **Saponins:** Found in potatoes, beans and grains. They boost the immune system and promote wound healing.

✦ **Capsaicin** seems to reduce the level of Substance P, a compound that contributes to inflammation and pain, and may inhibit cancer-generating substances. Found in peppers.

Food as more than sustenance

Food is comfort. Food is culture. Food is social. Food is art. Food is beauty. Food is sensory, pleasure and joy. In most cultures, eating is a sacred experience. *'When food is blessed by being shared, by being eaten in fellowship amidst conversation and laughter, all food is health food'* says medical health expert and author Dr Andrew Weil.

Food as pleasure

Dr Weil goes on to say that *'Eating well must embrace both the health-promoting and pleasure-giving aspects of food'*. There is no doubt that eating can be an intensely pleasurable experience. The joy of eating is about indulging the colours, textures and aromas as well as the taste of your food. Scientists believe they have discovered a pleasure pathway through your brain into your body. When these pathways are stimulated and travelled by pleasurable impulses – from satisfying experiences – substances are released into your body that enhance your immunity.

Professor David Warburton (Stanford University) and colleagues from 'Arise' (Associates for Research into the Science of Enjoyment), believe that even those so-called 'naughty ' pleasures, such as chocolate and cheesecake, in moderation can be beneficial, as long as they are unaccompanied by guilt. Guilt produces as many negative effects as pleasure does positives ones.

Family eating

Family mealtimes are tremendously important. It is the time that bonding and sharing can take place, for real connection as a family unit. Even though it may be noisy and boisterous, meals establish family rituals that become the glue that holds you together. This is the time that real communication can take place, ideas can be exchanged and support offered to a family member who is needing it. It is remarkable how few families sit together even once a week for a meal.

Although it is very difficult to establish regular mealtimes within a busy family, you should aim for a session or two a week. You may be a single parent, or both parents may have late schedules, young children and babies need to eat earlier and older children often have late extra-mural activities.

Notwithstanding your family's demanding schedule, you should make an effort to set aside at least a few dinner times a week where everyone sits together to eat.

Food as a cultural experience

Every culture has a rich tradition surrounding food and mealtimes. From births and coming of age to weddings and religious festivities, eating delicious food is central to the experience. Women (and some men, too) spend an enormous amount of time and energy preparing dishes based on centuries-old traditions. Wonderful spices, herbs and best quality fresh ingredients are lovingly transformed into celebrations. The food becomes a symbol of love, comfort, traditional connections to the past and spiritual connection to a heritage.

Conscious eating

It is easy to just go through the motions as you fill yourself with food from meal to meal. You are often not conscious of what you are eating, distracted by a million things other than the meal, or glued to the TV. To focus on your food with a sense of awareness and gratitude is a spiritual practice and also enhances your digestion.

Ideally you should try to eat in a quiet and settled atmosphere whenever possible. Encourage the rest of your family to do the same. However, with a large family and small children, dinner time may be chaotic. This is often true for me. The last thing I am able to do is focus on the 'colours, textures and aromas' of my plateful. I am usually dishing up at the same time as coaxing one or two mouthfuls of fish into a mouth that is moaning for Coco Pops.

I sometimes just wait a few moments until everyone seems settled and then eat in a more dignified manner. I rather try to turn my lunchtime (even a tuna salad or sandwich and tea at my work desk) into a quiet settled, pleasurable meal. Your emotions also affect your digestion. If you are angry, irritable and uptight, wait a while before you eat. Your digestive system mirrors your state of mind. Anger, tension and conflict interfere with your body's capacity to digest.

Comfort food

Food as a source of comfort is not always a bad thing. Think of the warm childhood memories around food. Feelings within you may be evoked by chicken soup, soft mielie pap, maltabella porridge, rice pudding or sweet tea. It may trigger memories of a loving parent or grandparent attending to your needs and nurturing you through difficult times.

The eating of comfort food at times is pleasurable and even beneficial. However, you need to be aware and conscious as you spoil yourself. Ask yourself a simple question '*Am I indulging in a simple comfort or am I feeding an addiction?*'

A thin slice of chocolate cake with a steaming cup of coffee fills an emotional need, but finishing the entire cake is probably due to a deeper hunger within you that food cannot satisfy. Comfort habits are comforting, addictions are serious.

If you feel that you eat sweet comfort foods very often and usually when you are not even hungry, or you cannot stop when you have had a single slice, you may need to address this issue. If you eat like this and are either significantly overweight or have seriously fluctuating weight, it is worth confronting the bigger issues that may be present. You may need to enrol in a few sessions with a counsellor to discuss any eating issues connected to your emotional or psychological health.

Before you grab a snack to eat, ask yourself whether the desire right now is for comfort or nourishment. Are you hungry or are you just responding to boredom, self-pity, depression or a habit?

If your answer is '*No, I am not really hungry*' then you have a choice to opt for an alternative. Rather go for a walk, perform a ten-minute breathing exercise, meditate, listen to beautiful music or even soak in a fragrant bathtub.

If you really feel like that chocolate chip cookie, take one or two on a plate with a cup of tea, enjoy it guiltlessly and then get on with whatever else you were doing. If you continually deprive yourself, you will obsess about that cookie until you finally rebel and eat the whole packet!

Food as medicine

'Let your Food be your Medicine and let your Medicine be your Food'
This concept espoused by Hippocrates, the father of medicine, 2000 years ago, has never been more topical than it is today. There is an ever-growing appreciation of the major role diet plays in determining your health. Nutrition is, to a large extent, accepted as a therapeutic healing modality. There is even something called 'Nutritional Medicine' which means the use of diet and supplements to aid in treating medical illnesses and conditions. Diet is always primary and supplementation (vitamins, etc) sec-

113

ondary. More and more research indicates that certain dietary practices cause as well as prevent a whole host of diseases. In addition to the nutritional value of food for energy supply and maintenance of body functioning, there are two important effects of food:
1. Damaging effects – Destructive to your health, potential for illness.
2. Healing value – value beyond energy and building blocks ('Food as medicine').

1. Damaging foodstuffs
You should certainly cut down on your intake of these foods, but it does not mean you have to eliminate them completely. If you go out for dinner or have friends over for a braai, enjoy your piece of steak, but do not do it too often. The same is true for your delicious cappuccino that you indulge in when you are out. Try to cut back during your work day on caffeine and rather choose to drink rooibos (red bush) or herbal teas and keep the coffee for a treat.

Table 5: Damaging foods

Food substances that are damaging	Found in these foods
Saturated fats	Pork, beef, lamb, poultry skin, cream and full-cream dairy products, coconut and palm kernel oil (found in many biscuits and baked goods).
Transfatty acids	Margarine, ready to bake potato chips, potato crisps, deep-fried foods, pastries.
Refined sugar	Sweets, chocolates, fizzy drinks, biscuits, bakery goods, some breakfast cereals.
Nitrates and nitrites	Smoked fish, smoked meat, cold cuts of meat, sausages, polony.
Pesticides	Sprayed onto almost all fruit and vegetables except organic produce. Wash all fruit and raw vegetables.
Food colouring	Sweets, coloured fizzy drinks, breakfast cereals, potato crisps.

Table 5: Damaging foods (continued)

Food substances that are damaging	Found in these foods
Food additives	Almost all tinned, frozen, smoked and processed foodstuffs. *(Increase your intake of fresh foods to counter this!)*
Excessive salt	Smoked foods, cold cuts of meat, sausages, polony, potato crisps.
Excessive caffeine	Coffee, cola drinks, chocolate.

2. Healing foods

Table 6: Healing foods

Healing food substances	Found in these foods	Action
Phytochemicals	Fruit and vegetables	See Table 4 on page 108.
Omega-3 fatty acids	Fatty fish – mackerel, salmon, sardines, herring – and walnuts	Excellent for hormone balance, cell function, joints, bones and mental function.
Omega-6 fatty acids	Found in most oils including sunflower oil	Protective effect on your heart and blood vessels.
Acidophilus – live bacterial culture	Good quality yoghurt	Strengthens immune system, aids digestion, may reduce incidence of some cancers and heart disease.
Good oils	Pumpkin, sunflower and sesame seeds	Lubricate joints and skin, help blood-clotting pathways, may aid in general healing.
Phyto-oestrogens	Soya beans	Possible protection against breast and prostate cancer.
Mono-unsaturated fats	Avocado, olive oil, macadamia nuts	May have cardio-protective effect.
Low GI carbs	See Table 1 on page 107	Great energy source with slow entry into bloodstream.
Fibre	Unpeeled fruit and vegetables, wholemeal or wholegrain cereal foods, pulses, oats	Aids intestinal transit, slows down the release of glucose into your bloodstream. May reduce risk of heart disease by reducing blood cholesterol.

Food and your hormones

When you hear the word hormone, you immediately think of PMT, menopause, pregnancy or sex. These sex hormones – oestrogen and in men testosterone – are just two sex hormones among hundreds of general body hormones.

Hormones regulate almost every function in your body, from controlling blood glucose levels to mechanisms such as the stress response, daily rhythms and growth and repair. The hormone pathways are known as the *endocrine system*. This is how the system works: Something causes a stimulus to a gland. This gland then sends a message in the form of a hormone into the bloodstream to reach an organ or more specifically a cell. The cell receives the message and then responds with an action that the messenger has ordered.

The pancreas is the gland that secretes the hormone insulin into the bloodstream. The insulin travels to the liver and to the muscles, telling them to take glucose from the blood and store it. The liver and muscle cells do just that. So when insulin levels increase, blood glucose levels will decrease (because the glucose has been stored in the liver and muscles). If the glucose levels fall too low, the brain (which requires glucose to function) calls out for more glucose. If the brain doesn't get more glucose, it starts to become less efficient. You may get dizzy, weak, blurry. You know this term as hypoglycemia (low blood sugar). So if you eat a huge carb pasta lunch, you will cause a huge surge of insulin, which pushes the glucose into storage and soon after your lunch you feel extremely fatigued.

Insulin does not function on its own. It has a 'partner' called glucagon, also secreted from the pancreas. While insulin drives blood sugar levels down (by putting them into storage), glucagon has the opposite effect. It increases blood glucose levels. By these two hormones working in unison, a tight control of glucose is maintained, allowing the brain to function at its best.

Insulin and carbohydrates

For many years you have been told to eat less fat and more carbohydrates. But for the past 15 years throughout the developed world, people have been eating less fat and getting fatter. Despite the dramatic cutback on fat consumption and the flood of 'lite' (i.e. lower fat) products, the paradox is that people are eating less fat and getting fatter. So a conclusion to reach is that perhaps a low-fat, high carb diet may be dangerous to your health. It is certainly important what you consume in the form of calories and amounts of fats, carbs and protein. But your body's hormonal response to food and what it does in its processing and metabolism of food is just as important (if not more so).

Your body requires a continual intake of carbohydrates (which are broken down into glucose) to feed your brain, which uses glucose as its main energy supply. Any carb not immediately used by your body will be stored in the form of glycogen. The body has two sites for storage – the liver and the muscles. Only the glycogen from the liver is able to be broken down and sent back into the bloodstream to be used by the brain. Your liver's glycogen stores can easily be depleted within 12 hours so it must maintain a continuous glycogen supply. Hence your need to eat carbs.

But what happens when you eat too much carbohydrate? The total storage capacity for carbohydrate is really quite limited. The average person can store about 350 grams of carbs in your muscles (which cannot be used by your brain) and about 60-90 grams in your liver (which is accessible for brain fuel). This is approximately equivalent to three slices of bread or two cups of pasta to keep the brain working.

Once this storage capacity in the liver and muscles is filled, excess carbohydrates have just one destination – to be converted into fat and stored. So even though carbs are fat-free, excess carbs end up as excess fat.

A high-carb meal will cause a quick rise in blood sugar, stimulating the pancreas to secrete insulin, lowering the blood glucose.

So in short, insulin is a storage hormone to convert excess carbs into fat (in case of future famine). So the insulin that is secreted by excess carb stimulus may promote body fat accumulation. Too much carb = too much insulin = 'fat storage'.

The key to all this is the SPEED at which carbohydrates enter the bloodstream because this speed determines the rate of insulin secretion. Whether you take in pasta, rice cakes, carrots, apples or sweets; they are

117

all broken down into simple glucose in the stomach and then absorbed into the bloodstream. All carbs enter at different rates. The entry rate of a carb into the bloodstream is the Glycaemic Index.

You now can understand the concept of GI with greater clarity. When a carb enters the bloodstream very fast, the pancreas responds by secreting a lot of insulin. Although that will now bring the blood sugar level down, it also sends a message to the body to store fat and keep it stored. So many very high GI carbs can not only make you fat, they can also keep you that way. So what can you do to modify this response?

Low GI carbohydrates
These low GI carbs have a very slow rate of entry into bloodstream, so do not cause as great a surge of insulin, and therefore are less likely to precipitate fat storage. They also make you feel full for longer.

Eat moderate amounts of protein with your carbs
This will slow the rate of glucose transit into your blood, as protein is broken down and digested. Protein is also a stimulus for the secretion from the pancreas of the hormone glucagon which has the opposite effect to insulin.

You are now aware how protein is an essential component in your body and is vital for the structure of your cells and immunity. So if protein is so crucial and if excess carbs can make you fat, why not eat lots of protein and very little carbs to lose weight? Low carb, high protein diets (see below) are the basis of many extremely popular quick weight loss programmes. Many of these diets say *'Eat as much protein as you want, and a lot of fat, as long as you don't eat many carbs!'*

Almost everyone will lose weight at first. But the problem is that these high-protein diets induce a state of 'ketosis'. This happens when you have inadequate amounts of glycogen in the liver to meet the needs of your body (especially your brain). The body uses fat to supply this fuel. Doesn't that sound great! 'Fat burning' is what you want!

The problem is that the conversion of fat into energy gets short-circuited. As a result, your cells produce abnormal chemicals called *ketone bodies*. The body has no use for these ketone bodies and tries like crazy to get rid of them through your urine. That equals a lot of weight loss at first, mainly in the form of water. And what you may not know is that the excess protein at each meal means excess conversion of the protein that you do not need into fat! Over 90 per cent of people who lose weight on very high protein, low-carb ketogenic diets put on all their weight again. Some research shows that the actual fat cells may change, making them up to ten times more active in fat than before the diet.

Exercise

Exercise is also a modulator of your hormones. Regular exercise will reduce your insulin levels and increase your levels of glucagon. This helps with breakdown rather than storage of fat.

Weight loss and diets

The problems with diets are manifold. All of the different diets will work for a while but then many result in a regaining of the 'lost' weight. A diet is impossible to stick to on a long-term basis. They set up all kinds of emotional responses that are not compatible with healthy living such as guilt, shame, feelings of deprivation and frustration. But in reality, most women at some stage of their lives (or most of the time) put themselves on a diet. Some are genuinely overweight. Others may need to lose a few kilos after a pregnancy or a holiday, while the vast majority are in continual pursuit of the 'elusive' slimmer body!

Being very overweight or indeed obese are serious health hazards and must be tackled with a comprehensive weight loss programme. This should include a most favourable eating plan together with exercise and an approach to mental wellbeing. But, just as the common cold is never going to be wiped off the earth, so too are diets here to stay!

If weight loss alone is your goal regardless of any health risk, then you can certainly use any diet and you will lose weight. No one diet can guarantee that you will keep the extra weight off, but stick rigidly to any of the current diets and you are sure to lose kilos.

If you want to lose kilos and centimetres because you are indeed overweight, or you want to get back into a decent shape and look and feel

119

good but want optimal long-term health at the same time, then follow a responsible nutrition programme.

In this section I present to you a clinical review of all the current diet choices plus my own opinion on them. And then I outline the principles of the SELF diet to help lose that unwanted flab and stay in tip-top, glowing health!

It is most important that you have as much knowledge as possible so you can make wise decisions. One of the most controversial debates at the moment is the popularity of high protein diets with very low or no carb content. Too much of the wrong high GI carbs are certainly no good. The backlash to this has been a blanket ban of all carbs in certain diets, This ban on all carbs has meant disposing of essential nutrients in fruits, vegetables, pulses and fibre-rich grains. The backlash has also brought about a dramatic increase in proteins including harmful, fatty, damaging foods.

Debate about no-carb/(very low carb) and high protein diets.
Supporters of low-carb diets (e.g. Atkins Diet, Zone Diet, South Beach Diet) say that carb-cravings and associated conditions like insulin-resistance, unstable blood-glucose levels and obesity levels are the result of overconsumption of carbs, especially refined carbohydrates. While the connection between excessive consumption of refined carbs and ill-health is now well documented, there is considerable controversy about the nutritional status of unrefined carbs or low Glycemic Index carbs. At present, most nutritionists and dietitians regard these 'good carbs' as essential to good diet nutrition. Also, second generation lower-carb diets, like the South Beach Diet, are moving towards a diet plan which includes more carbs.

The different diets: What works? What's in? What's out?
Of the many different diet approaches, all have some value and most will ensure that you do lose weight. There is no one perfect plan. The importance is for you to have as much information as possible to make an informed decision according to your lifestyle. Please note that much of

Why high-protein, low-carb diets may not be for you:

1. They do not represent nutritionally balanced eating. For some dieters, these diets can be harmful.

2. Some popular high-protein diet foods may be high in cholesterol and saturated fat, which are now established as major culprits in heart attacks and strokes.

3. Some protein diets may overload you with protein, which results in loss of calcium from your bones, which may lead to osteoporosis. Protein overload also stresses your kidneys as they eliminate large amounts of urea, a by-product of protein metabolism.

4. They forbid foods known to lower the risk of heart disease and many cancers.

5. They restrict carbohydrates, the nutrient group most readily converted to energy. Even moderately active people will notice this lack during exercise.

6. They deprive your brain of glucose, which it needs for normal functioning. The result may be a slow down in thinking and reaction time.

7. They deprive you of the enormous benefits of fibre, which is a form of carbohydrate (cellulose).

8. They may be deficient in essential vitamins. Indeed, some high-protein diets even require you to take vitamin supplements for the sake of your health.

9. They cause potentially dangerous changes in your body chemistry.

10. They deliver temporary weight loss, but a large part of it is water weight and lean muscle mass – not fat. (You lose water because your kidneys get rid of the excess waste products of protein and fat, called ketones.)

my comment on these different programmes is based on medical and scientific data as well as *my own opinion and approach* to optimal health-care and lifestyle.

1. Diets with very high protein and extremely low carbohydrates

These diets claim you can eat all the protein and fat that you care to and still lose weight. All you need to do is simply cut out carbohydrates to become thin. This sounds so easy that when you first begin this type of diet, you cut out almost all carbohydrates except for a few vegies, but you can eat sour cream and steak and eggs. This will put your body into a state known as 'ketosis'. Many doctors agree that ketosis is an abnormal and unhealthy state with possible damaging effects to kidneys. The Dr Atkins Diet is probably the most well-known extremely low-carb/high-protein diet.

After stating on National Television that I did not approve of this kind of diet, I was challenged to at least try it. I did this for four weeks during the December holidays! I lost four kilos which I could not maintain when I simply began eating reasonably normally again. But I felt nauseous, lethargic and dizzy throughout the diet, even following a hearty meal of steak and eggs!

While there are countless success stories of people using this kind of diet, many found that they couldn't get through the beginning phase because they didn't feel well eating like this.

Advantages

+ You will lose weight fast.
+ You can eat large amounts of protein and still lose weight.
+ You eat very little sugar and white flour.

Drawbacks

+ Initial weight loss may be quite fast, but is not always sustainable.
+ A ketosis-inducing diet may strain the kidneys.
+ As many foods high in animal protein may also be high in saturated fat, your saturated fat intake may be too high for comfort.

My opinion

+ I am not keen to recommend such a restrictive low-carb/high-protein diet. It restricts healthy foods that provide essential nutrients and doesn't provide the variety of foods needed to meet nutritional needs adequately. If you remain on this diet for extended periods, you may be at risk for inadequate vitamin and mineral intake as well as more potential health risks.
+ For severely obese individuals, the cardiovascular risks of a high-protein diet may be worth taking in order to reduce the extra, well-documented risks of severe obesity. However, this issue is outside the

scope of this review and should be settled between yourself and your doctor. If you are not seriously obese, I do not recommend the more restrictive type of low-carb/high-protein diet plan.

2. Low carbs, moderate protein diets

On this kind of diet you eat normal-sized helpings of lean meats, such as skinless chicken and turkey, as well as fish and shellfish. Vegetables are also allowed, as are nuts, low-fat cheese and eggs, legumes, canola and olive oils. The goal is to eat three balanced meals a day, and to eat enough so that you don't feel hungry all the time. You should avoid high-carb vegetables and fruits as well as many starches. You do slowly reintroduce some low GI carbs and good oils. An example is the popular South Beach Diet.

Advantages
+ Promotes good weight loss, rapid in the beginning (without many carbs).
+ Helps to improve eating habits and stabilise blood sugar levels.
+ Helps to improve good to bad cholesterol ratio and reduce triglycerides.

Drawbacks
Much of the initial weight loss is likely to be water weight loss caused by carbohydrate restriction. Such weight loss is typically regained, as soon as carb intake resumes.
+ This type of diet allows very little complex carbohydrates. Most of the world thrives on complex carbs and these foods do not keep you overweight, nor do they warrant such severe restrictions. These diets may perpetuate the current fear of carbs.
+ Low-carb diet plans are not generally recommended for anyone with kidney problems.

My opinion
Although I do not agree with some of the propositions in this kind of diet, it is far healthier than a very high-protein diet and is more balanced eating.

3. Hormonal (insulin control) -based diets

This type of diet is more focused on hormones than calories. It is based on how your body's hormones (essentially insulin and glucagon) respond to food. The premise is that the hormonal response and metabolism of food is as important, if not more so, than counting calories. The original diet plan with this philosophy is the Zone Diet, which promotes a 40-30-30 diet plan: 40 % carbohydrates, 30 % fat and 30 % protein at each meal.

Advantages
+ Very organised food plan.
+ Steady weight loss if followed exactly.
+ Valid scientific approach.

Drawbacks
+ Too scientific to be user-friendly.
+ You can't feed your family the same thing, because they have different calculations.
+ Time-consuming because you must eat six times each day.

My opinion
From my perspective as a doctor, I find the science of this approach enjoyable and it makes a lot of sense, but I do think at times it gets overwhelming. I did try the Zone Diet for a while and felt quite good on it. I felt strong with my exercise and was seldom hungry. The problem was that I did not lose much weight. We are all very different and it may work for you. For me the 40 per cent carbs was a little high. (My SELF diet contains slightly fewer carbs and a reduction of the fats at the beginning of the diet.) The hormonal control of food, particularly your sugar control, is very important as a principle on your eating plan. If you like a strict structure in your diet, then by all means try this type of diet.

4. Diet according to your genetics

The concept of genetically individualised nutrition has been introduced in recent times. The basis for this kind of diet is that as a result of certain genetic differences, each person digests and processes certain foods better than others. This concept is not generally accepted in scientific thinking as it is not supported by enough mainstream research. However, many people who have tried this diet claim that not only do they achieve their ideal weight, but very often many of their symptoms of ill-health clear up as well.

The first of this kind of diet is the Blood Group Diet. On each red blood cell we have a type of molecule that determines our main ABO blood group – A, AB, B or O. *(There are other markers on the blood cell that make a person Rhesus positive or negative.)* According to American Naturopath Dr Peter D'Adamo, each blood group has a different protocol to follow for nutrition and maximising health.

Advantages
✦ It is a popular way of following an individualised dietary program. You avoid certain foods apparently not digested well by your blood group and eat those recommended.
✦ Many people claim to feel better on this programme.

My opinion
✦ If we are to settle on blood groups as important to the food we should eat, why confine ourselves to the ABO blood type system? There is another system called Rhesus blood grouping and there are a vast number of antigens on our cells other than blood that are just as critically important as ABO antigens.
✦ I find that a lot of the food that is either recommended for my blood group is not the kind of food I choose to eat. I do not enjoy a lot of red meat and poultry. It also recommends a high-carbohydrate low-fat diet – which doesn't work for me – and tells me to avoid dairy, which I enjoy and find nutritious in small amounts.

5. Food Combining Diets
There are several food-combining diets on the market:

In order to optimise your digestion and weight loss, you should avoid eating certain foods as part of the same meal. For example, you should not eat carbohydrates with proteins. Some versions advocate eating only fruit or fruit juices before noon. Most advocate starting out eating only fruit. Thereafter, vegetables and a small amount of starch. Some food combining plans permit 'sweet-allowances' and others don't, and some insist on waiting four hours between protein meals and starch meals.

Advantages
✦ A food combining diet may benefit you for a couple of days, as a type of 'detox' diet.
✦ Also, due to the very low-calorie nature of the early stages of the diet, weight loss is virtually assured.

Drawbacks
✦ There is no hard scientific evidence to support the idea that weight loss becomes more likely if you separate certain foods. Also, they may fall below minimum recommended calorie levels.

My opinon
If you feel good by eating fruit and raw vegetables for a day or two, there is no harm. There is also no harm choosing to eat your starch at a different meal from your protein if you like this kind of plan. Your body is designed to digest the different food groups all at the same time, so it does not make much scientific sense to me, but there is very little harm involved.

The final verdict
There is none! The last word on diet is not yet out and the controversy will continue. My advice is – do not believe anyone who tells you *'this is the only way, the ultimate truth!'* with regard to your diet, healing or any aspect of your life. Many paths have value. Look for the honest and the authentic that rings true for you and your life (and a little bit of science always helps!).

There is no doubt that if you cut back on your intake of calories, you will lose weight. Any diet will work; even bananas and cream three times a day! The two questions you need to ask yourself are:

1. Is this diet and the concurrent loss of weight sustainable?
2. Is it healthy for me in the long term?

An interesting spin on diets and eating plans (with which I agree) is expressed by Dr Andrew Weil. He suggests that the reason people do so well (even healing takes place) when embarking on a new eating plan is the associated shift in consciousness that occurs, together with the decision to embark on the programme now. The mental resolution to 'do it now' results in a most positive outcome. And I believe that the greater the mental and emotional resolve, the more powerful the effects.

SELF diet

My diet, which is entitled the SELF diet following the title of this book, is based on the six principles of this book (plus three more concepts). I do not make claims to miracle cures and enormous, quick weight loss results.

The SELF diet places the power of health and energy and effective nutrition and even weight loss in your hands by giving you all the facts. It cuts through the hype and confusion and gives you responsible information based on credible science. It also extends the power of eating, diets and nutrition beyond your body to the multifaceted person you are – your beauty, your ageing, your bones, your vanity, your insecurities, your depression , your moods, your lifestyle, your whole life.

Yes, women still do want to be told what to eat. I know this as fact as I too have consulted the experts time and again.

So I will not disappoint you – the SELF diet has a section at the end of the chapter of *what to eat*. This is a programme aimed at recharging your energy and your life.

1. Empower

Take charge of your body and your diet. The SELF diet means YOU make the decisions. You do not hand over control to a dietician or doctor. They are simply there to guide you. Empowerment means knowledge. Gain clear and responsible information so that you have the power to make good choices.

2. Embrace

The SELF diet requires that you begin to embrace your body, your femininity and your beauty. You need to let go of self-loathing and learn to appreciate the gift of your body, even when it means coming to terms with its limitations. I am a tall, large-framed woman and will never be petite! A crucial step in this weight loss programme is to be realistic. The SELF diet ensures that your eating helps to maintain primarily your health as well as your beauty, your skin quality and anti-ageing and to be the best you can at each stage. The SELF diet means you get a grip on your emotions, too. If you are carrying many emotional issues that are causing you distress, and you are depressed, anxious or miserable, this will interfere with your loss of weight.

3. Eat

Diet is not starvation. Watch calories, watch quantities, watch hormones but eat . . . you need to kick-start your metabolism. Starvation blunts your metabolism and you cannot lose weight. Eat but eat less – any caloric restriction will help you lose. You need to restrict calories healthily! This means eat *nutrient-dense food* instead of calorie-dense food. For example, substitute fat-free milk in place of low-fat or full-cream products. Eat a vegetable dish full of colourful green and orange veggies with fresh tomatoes and herbs instead of potatoes and rice with your meal.

4. Exercise

On the SELF diet you *have* to exercise! And that means frequently and for extended periods. No quick fix here. A 30-minute sweat at the gym three times a week just doesn't facilitate weight loss. Try to get to four to five sessions of endurance i.e. power-walking or swimming for up to 45-60 minutes at a time.

5. Energy

Food is a source of energy. It is your fuel. Use the freshest, highest quality *energising* fuel/foodstuffs. Plenty of salads, soups, raw and cooked vegetables and fresh fruit are the centre of the SELF diet.

6. Enrich
Weight loss is not only a body thing. If you are feeling lonely, discon-nected and without a sense of spiritual wellbeing, you will not manage to lose weight easily. You need to enrich your life and your body.

Plus three more . . .

1. Equilibrium
It is all about balance. The SELF diet is not about HIGH anything! Not high proteins, not high fats and not high carbs. It is about a balance/equili-brium of moderate protein, moderate carbs and moderate fats. According to most diet experts, the best diet is a balanced eating plan, low in satu-rated fat and refined sugar, and moderate in all the food groups But remember BEST quality, MODERATE quantity.

2. Excellence
The SELF diet means excellent food choices: excellent proteins (fish and plant), excellent carbs (low GI) and excellent fats (mono-unsaturates).

3. Ease
To *lose weight* and *gain health* at the same time is NOT complicated and does NOT create a difficult lifestyle. You should not have to fret with things like weighing your foods and fussing around meals. Your life includes eat-ing out – at friends, in restaurants, while travelling and on the run (where most women are most of the time!). The SELF diet should bring you to a place of 'ease'. Your motto on the SELF diet should be *'Easy does it'*.

Should women supplement?
While anyone worth her weight in nutrition credentials will advise women to first turn to food for their nutrition needs, in reality many women don't get enough nutrients in their daily diet from food alone. Ideally, a healthy diet including all the food groups and plenty of fresh fruit and vegetables should contribute all your mineral and vitamin requirements. In the real world, where women diet, skip meals or eat on

the run, all while juggling work demands and a family, you are probably not getting all the nutrients you require from your diet. Approximately one half of middle-aged women do not consume even two-thirds of the recommended amounts of many vitamins.

The term *nutritional supplementation* includes the use of vitamins, minerals and other food factors supporting good health, and preventing or helping treat illnesses. Their role is primarily as components of enzymes.

Growing numbers of people worldwide are taking supplements. Despite the tremendous body of research supporting the use of nutritional supplementation, most medical experts have still not publicly endorsed supplementation, even though 80 per cent of them take supplements themselves!

Numerous studies have demonstrated that most women consume a diet inadequate in nutritional value. The level of deficiency is not usually severe enough to result in obvious signs and symptoms. A severe deficiency disease like scurvy (lack of vitamin C) is extremely rare but marginal vitamin C deficiency appears to be relatively common. In many instances the only clue of a nutrient deficiency may be fatigue, difficulty in concentration or a non-specific feeling of being unwell. Marginal dietary intake is linked to many mental, emotional and physical problems, including memory loss, mood swings, depression, irritability or osteoporosis. Taking a moderate-dose multivitamin and mineral supplement that contains extra vitamin E, plus a second supplement of calcium and magnesium, for example, will help provide nutritional insurance.

The RDAs are based on scientific research of both humans and animals and are set at levels to provide for 98 per cent of healthy people. These guidelines were originally developed to reduce the rates of severe nutritional deficiencies such as scurvy (vitamin C deficiency), pellagra (niacin deficiency) and beriberi (vitamin B1 deficiency), not to promote optimal health! Another problem is that they were designed to serve as the basis for evaluating the adequacy of whole groups of populations, not individuals. Finally, the RDAs were designed for normal healthy people (as far back as 1941), not those experiencing unusual stressors in 2005. A tremendous amount of scientific research indicates that the 'optimal' level for certain nutrients, especially the antioxidants such as vitamin C and E, betacarotene and selenium, may be much higher than their current RDAs.

The RDAs do not take into account environmental and lifestyle factors which can destroy vitamins and bind to minerals. For example, even the International Food and Nutrition Boards acknowledge that smokers require at least twice the amount of vitamin C as non-smokers. But effects of alcohol consumption, food additives, heavy metals, carbon monoxide fumes, pesticides and other chemicals in our 21st-century environment are not considered.

In addition to essential nutrients, there are other food components and natural agents which have demonstrated impressive health-promoting effects. Examples of these include carotenoids, flavonoids, probiotics, carnitine and coenzyme Q10 (see Phytochemicals on page 107). These compounds exert significant therapeutic effects with little if any toxicity. More and more research indicates that these accessory nutrients, although not considered essential in the classical sense, may play a huge role in preventing illness. (Office of Dietary Supplements, National Institute of Health, Bethesda, Maryland.

Vitamin A
The RDA is 800 to 1000 IU. Vitamin A has a role in vision, the adaptation to light and dark. It is important in skeletal and soft tissue growth and in the reproductive function. Beta-carotene, a precursor of vitamin A, is the pigment in fruit and vegetables and supplies about $2/3$ of the vitamin supply in human nutrition. Several anticancer properties of beta-carotene have been reported. Orange or yellow vegetables, such as carrots and green leafy vegetables, are generally good sources of this important antioxidant. If taken as a supplement, current information indicates it may be best to use mixed carotenoids from natural sources rather than synthetic fl-carotene.

The B vitamins
They are important during stress, for helping fight disease, and especially for obtaining energy from proteins, fats and carbohydrates. Sex, alcohol,

Table 7 Supplements

(Note: Recommended doses are for women age 25-60)

Supplement	Required for	In larger doses
Vitamin A	Reproduction, vision, maintenance of skin and linings of organs.	May be important in cancer prevention
Beta-carotene	Is a source of vitamin A	Protect against cancers, antioxidant effect and anti-carcinogenesis
Vitamin D	Bone maintenance, helps absorption of calcium	You do not want vitamin D in large doses as it can be toxic.
Vitamin E	Protects cell membranes from oxidative damage	Protects against cancer, infection resistance and boosts immunity
Vitamin C	Immunity, collagen formation, bone maintenance	May protect against cancer, cardiovascular and cerebro-vascular disease, prevent cataracts, protect respiratory tract from infections
Vitamin B12	Essential for central nervous system function	No need for high doses
Folate/Folic acid	Essential for red blood cells; also now shown importance in prevention heart disease, stroke, cancer and fetal neural tube defects	Prevention of birth defects and heart disease
Vitamin B6 (Pyridoxine)	Growth and maintenance of almost every body function	Supplementation may help carpal tunnel syndrome, PMS and nerve problems
Vitamin B1 (Thiamine)	Needed for metabolic functions	No need or benefit in high doses
Vitamin B2-Riboflavin	Required for tissue repair, vision and blood	May help with ageing, especially preventing cataracts
Calcium	Required for bone structure, energy production, and nerve communication	Not ideal to take more than 1200 mg
Magnesium	Many metabolic functions	Possible antioxidant effect (neutralises damaged cells)
Selenium	Antioxidant function	Antioxidant function protective against certain cancers and tumors

Possible toxicity	RDA	Optimal health dose	Found in
Can cause toxicity (most serious – birth defects)	800 mg	200 mg	Vitamin A (carotenoids) abundant in darkly coloured fruits and vegetables. Also certain foodstuffs such as breakfast cereals and milk also provide it.
Not at all toxic	n/a	80 mg	Orange or yellow vegetables, green leafy vegetables
Can be toxic at high levels	5 mg	18 mg	Sunlight UV exposure (will not cause toxicity)
Very safe in high doses except not to be used for people on anticoagulant therapy.	8 mg	400 mg	Wheatgerm, the oils of grains, leafy greens, various seeds and beans.
Generally no toxic effects; in very high doses may cause diarrhoea or very rarely kidney stones	60 mg	400 mg	Fresh fruit esp. citrus and kiwi fruit leafy greens, and vegetables
Safe but rarely needed as supplement	2 mg	2 mg	Meat products and to lesser extent egg yolk, milk
Safe even at high levels	180 mg	1000 mg	Beef, liver, spinach, beans, fortified foods, broccoli, avocado, asparagus
Very high doses may cause problems – sensory and motor impairments	1.6 mg	10 mg	Wheatgerm and bran, beans, meat, poultry, fish, and some fruits and vegetables
Harmless in high levels, few reports of gastric upset	1.1 mg	7 mg	Beans, peas, leafy green vegetables, milk, beef and liver
No known toxicity	1.3 mg	2 mg	Beans, peas, leafy green vegetables, milk, beef and liver
Not toxic, but not ideal to take beyond 1200 mg	800-200 mg	800-1200 mg	Dairy products, seeds and leafy vegetables
Non-toxic	280 mg	450 mg	Nuts, vegetables, brown rice, parsley, spinach and other leafy greens.
Probably non-toxic	55 mg	150 mg	Green vegetables

sun exposure and stress use up the B vitamins. There are eight B vitamins but three of the major ones are thiamin, riboflavin and niacin. While some of the B vitamins are produced by your gut flora, you also get some from your food. The germ and bran parts of cereals are good sources of B vitamins, as are beans, peas, leafy green vegetables, milk, beef and liver. Vegetarian diets are often poor sources of B vitamins.

Vitamin C
It is also known as ascorbic acid or ascorbate. It is the most important of the water soluble antioxidants, and is important for coping with disease and stress. Vitamin C helps spare other antioxidants such as glutathione and vitamin E, and is required by the immune system. Fresh fruit, leafy greens and vegetables are sources.

Vitamin E
It is another fat-soluble antioxidant. It is important for lung function, blood circulation, protection against free radical (oxidation) damage, and membrane function. Natural forms have been shown to be better than synthetic forms. In your food, sources of vitamin E are wheat germ, the oils of grains, leafy greens, various seeds and beans.

Important minerals
Selenium
Selenium, a metal, is an important antioxidant. It's required in only tiny amounts. High levels are poisonous. From food sources, you will not get toxic levels. Good food sources depend on their geographic origin. It is a good idea to make sure your multivitamin contains 50 micrograms.

Zinc and copper
These are needed by many enzymes, including those in your stomach, intestines and the immune system. Sources of zinc are seafood, sunflower and pumpkin seeds, mushrooms, spinach and soybeans. Sources of copper are wholegrains, leafy greens, cherries, vegetables, nuts, eggs, fish and poultry dark meats. The food we eat supplies about 15 mg of zinc per day.

Magnesium and calcium
They are needed by the body, for keeping bones healthy. Calcium is high in dairy products, seeds and leafy vegetables. Magnesium is high in nuts, vegetables, brown rice, parsley, spinach and other leafy greens. The RDA for calcium is 800 mg a day. Calcium is important in bone formation, tooth formation, blood clotting, nerve transmission, muscle contraction and relaxation and enzyme activation.

Iron
The RDA is 10 to 15 mg per day. Iron is an important part of haemoglobin formation. Haemoglobin is the part of your blood that transports oxygen. Iron is also very important during growth and pregnancy.

Superfoods?
So although taking a mega- or multivitamin/mineral and extra antioxidants is part of a good health promoting and longevity strategy, there is NO substitute for including a generous amount of a variety of the above 'Super Foods' in our diets.

Nutrition, women and special needs
Diet and pregnancy
If your diet is balanced and not too heavy in sugar or fat, you don't need to change the way you eat dramatically during your pregnancy.

It is very common to experience morning sickness during the first trimester. If you are experiencing this nausea and are unable to eat a well-balanced diet, you may wonder whether or not you are getting enough nutrition for you and the baby. The fact is you can go for several weeks not eating an optimal diet without any ill effects on the baby. You may find that the only foods you can tolerate are carbohydrate-dense foods. If all you feel like eating is pasta and bread, then do not worry. It is more important that you keep something down rather than starve.

As the pregnancy progresses through the second and third trimester, you will feel better and be able to eat a wide range of nutritious foodstuffs. You will also slightly increase your intake of calories each day. The key is to make sure that your extra calories are packed with nutrients, protein, and good quality low GI carbohydrates.

The most important food group for you are fruits and vegetables as well as the high-fibre grains. These should be complemented with good proteins, such as fish and pulses, as well as moderate amounts of poultry and red meat. Your fat intake should once again be of the best quality olive oils, avocados and nuts.

You will certainly gain weight during your pregnancy but there should be a balanced approach to this. An excessive weight gain is extremely unhealthy and very difficult to lose after the birth, but an insufficient diet and intense weight management during pregnancy is unhealthy for the mother and especially for the baby.

Diet and menopause

Weight gain: This is often a problem after menopause. There is a slowing of metabolism and with each decade it is common to gain a few kilograms. Hormone therapy may also increase your appetite. In addition, postmenopausal women's figures begin to change as they gain more weight above the belt. As your abdominal girth increases, so does your risk of illnesses such as diabetes, high blood pressure and heart disease. Therefore if you are overweight especially across your abdominal region, you may want to consider losing as little as 10 per cent of your body weight to significantly reduce your disease risk.

Soya: Hot flushes are the hallmark of menopause for many women. Estrogen-like compounds, called phytoestrogens, found in soybeans can help offset this drop in estrogen. While not exactly like estrogen, phyto-estrogens act much like the female hormone, binding to the body's estrogen receptors and supplementing the effects of estrogen when levels are low. Studies report that hot flushes can be reduced by up to 40 per cent when women add soya to their diets. But how much is enough? Preliminary evidence suggests that about two cups of soy milk or a small amount of tofu daily might be all a woman needs to help dampen the hot flush and curb the estrogen swells during menopause.

Mood food: As hormones fluctuate, so does brain chemistry, including a powerful nerve chemical called serotonin. Peri- and postmenopausal women who struggle with mild depression might have lower serotonin levels than other women. While low levels of the chemical may cause a woman to crave sweets and feel grumpy, an increase in serotonin turns off the cravings and restores a more agreeable mood. If serotonin is at the root of the mood swings, then including a carbohydrate-rich, low GI snack could be all it takes to boost serotonin levels and mood. Be sure to eat the low GI variety.

Calcium: During and after menopause, you face a higher risk of osteoporosis. Women who consume ample calcium throughout life enter menopause with strong bones and are at lower risk of developing osteoporosis. Unfortunately, most women don't get enough calcium. In fact, one out of every two postmenopausal women consumes less than half the recommended calcium allotment (1200mg to 1500mg) needed to prevent age-related bone loss. Non-fat milk or calcium and vitamin D fortified soya milk are good sources of calcium and vitamin D, a nutrient essential for transporting calcium into the bones. It is best to take a supplement that contains 500mg of calcium.

Heart smart through menopause: Your risk for heart disease escalates quickly as estrogen levels drop after menopause. Hormone replacement therapy, diet and exercise can significantly reduce heart disease risk. Adopting a low-fat, high-fibre diet that includes a wide range of fresh fruits and vegetables, wholegrain breads and cereals, legumes including soybeans and non-fat dairy products, can help keep blood-fat levels low and heart disease at bay.

Nutrition and ageing

Physiological changes occur slowly over time in all your body systems. These changes are influenced by your life events, illnesses, genetic traits and socioeconomic factors. Nutrition remains important throughout your life, and even more so as you age. Many chronic diseases that develop later in life, such as osteoporosis, can be influenced by earlier poor dietary habits. But good nutrition in your later years still can help lessen the effects of diseases prevalent among older people or improve your quality of life. Poor nutrition, on the other hand, can prolong recovery from illnesses or worsen existing conditions. They include osteoporosis, obesity, high blood pressure, heart disease, certain cancers and gastrointestinal problems.

Studies show that a good diet in your later years helps both in reducing the risk of these diseases and in augmenting your body's healing capacity. This contributes to a higher quality of life.

As you age, you lose lean body mass. Reduced muscle mass includes skeletal muscle, smooth muscle and muscle that affects vital organ function, with loss of cardiac muscle perhaps the most important. Cardiac capacity can be reduced and cardiac function impaired by chronic diseases such as atherosclerosis, hypertension or diabetes. Changes also occur in the kidneys, lungs and liver, and in your ability to generate new protein tissue. In addition, ageing can slow the immune system's response in making antibodies. The most significant result of the loss of lean body mass may be the decrease in basal energy metabolism. Metabolic rate declines proportionately with the decline in total protein tissue. To avoid gaining weight, you must reduce calorie intake or increase activity. The goal is energy balance.

Total body fat typically increases with age. This often can be explained by too many calories. As you age, fat tends to concentrate in your trunk and especially fatty deposits around the vital organs. An enormous amount of new research has demonstrated that a calorie restricted diet is strongly associated with longevity. So don't starve yourself, but if you want to live longer cut down calorie intake!

Finally, you lose bone density with ageing. After menopause, women tend to lose bone mass at an accelerated rate. Recent attention has focused on the high incidence of osteoporosis. Severe osteoporosis is debilitating and serious. Fractures and their associated illness and mortality are certainly a significant concern. So do look after your bones! *Exercise, calcium and a good diet are essential throughout life.*

Nutrition is an important factor in all of the changes noted above i.e. loss of muscle mass, loss of bone density and increased body fat. However, the slowing of the normal action of the digestive tract also affects your total body function. Adequate dietary fibre, as opposed to increased use of laxatives, will maintain your regular bowel function and not interfere with the digestion and absorption of nutrients, as occurs with laxative use or abuse.

Your calorie needs change due to more body fat and less lean muscle. The challenge for the elderly is to meet the same nutrient needs as when you were younger, yet consume fewer calories. The answer to this problem is to choose foods high in nutrients in relation to their calories. Such foods are considered *'nutrient-dense'*. For example, low-fat milk is more nutrient dense than full-cream milk. Its nutrient content is the same, but it has fewer calories because it has less fat. Reducing the overall fat content in your diet is reasonable. It is the easiest way to cut calories. This is appropriate to reduce weight. Lower fat intake is often necessary because of chronic disease.

About 60 per cent of calories should come from carbohydrates, with emphasis on complex or low GI carbs. Complex carbohydrates put less stress on the circulating blood glucose than do refined carbohydrates.

Such a regime also enhances dietary fibre intake. Adequate fibre, together with adequate fluid, helps maintain normal bowel function. Fibre also is thought to decrease risk of intestinal inflammation. Vegetables, fruits, grain products, cereals, seeds, legumes and nuts are all sources of dietary fibre.

Your protein needs usually do not change although research studies are not definitive. Protein absorption may decrease as you age, and your body may make less protein. However, this does not mean protein intake should be routinely increased, because of the general decline in kidney function.

Vitamin deficiencies may not be obvious in many older people. However, any illness stresses the body and may be enough to use up whatever stores there are and make you vitamin deficient. Medications also interfere with many vitamins. So check out with your doctor whether any medication you may be taking is interfering. Although you may be cutting down on calories, your vitamin and mineral needs remain high.

Zinc, along with vitamins C and E, and the phytochemicals lutein, zeaxanthin and beta-carotene, may help prevent or slow the onset of age-related macular degeneration. The best way to obtain these nutrients is to consume at least five servings of fruits and vegetables, especially dark green, orange and yellow ones. Good choices include kale, spinach, broccoli, peas, oranges and spanspek (sweet melon). Consult your doctor to see if a supplement may also be necessary.

Vitamin E may have a potential role in the prevention of Alzheimer's disease. Research has shown that eating foods with vitamin E, like wholegrains, peanuts, nuts, vegetable oils and seeds, may help reduce the risk of Alzheimer's disease. However, the same benefits did not hold true from vitamin E supplements.

Low levels of vitamin B12 have been associated with memory loss and linked to age-related hearing loss in older adults. As we age, the amount of the chemical in the body needed to absorb vitamin B12 decreases. To avoid deficiency, older adults are advised to eat foods rich in vitamin B12 regularly, including meat, poultry, fish, eggs and dairy foods. Consult your doctor to see if a vitamin B12 supplement may also be necessary. and ask him or her to check your iron and calcium, too.

Chronic diseases of lifestyle, diabetes and diet

When it comes to heart disease and chronic diseases of lifestyle, the war on hypertension and high blood pressure (mainly through the use of medication) has resulted in a decrease in blood pressure and cholesterol but has not improved overall mortality. But the battle against the major risk factor – obesity and its frequent counterpart, Type II diabetes – has been totally lost! If you are overweight you should be concerned not only about the excess fat but rather the location of the fat. If it is around your abdomen, your risk for a heart attack is dramatically increased. This abdominal obesity usually indicates that you have a high level of insulin and are perhaps even predisposed to Type II diabetes. This is also known as adult onset diabetes, because it generally occurs after age 40 and accounts for almost 90 per cent of the diabetes population. Ironically, even though the insulin level is high, you may be on medication that further increases your insulin.

What often happens is that the cells become much less responsive to the insulin. More and more insulin is produced to try and reduce blood sugar levels.

The best way to try and treat Type II diabetes is to target excess body fat. Losing body fat has such a dramatic impact, not only on the diabetes and insulin control, but also on all the risk factors for a heart attack – the blood pressure, and the high cholesterol too. Unfortunately diets repeatedly fail!

You need to follow the principles of the SELF diet with the major focus on exercise (four to five times per week, for 45-60 minutes per session at a low intensity) and eating less calories ('nutrient-dense' rather than 'calorie-dense' food). A vital aspect of your eating programme is to slow the entry of glucose into your bloodstream. This means cutting out all high GI carbs. Eat small to moderate portions of low GI carbs together with moderate low-fat, good quality proteins. Restrict your fat intake but still add a restricted amount of good oils e.g. one half of an avocado or two teaspooons of olive oil thrown into your salads per day. You have to reduce your calorie intake. Sure, there is a hormonal regulation of your body but you need to eat less. Your levels of insulin will decrease and the size and mass of your fat cells will actually shrink. Your levels of cholesterol and fats (triglycerides) will be lowered and thereby help keep open your heart's vital vessels.

Remember your health is in your hands. Your good diet and lifestyle choices may determine to a large extent whether your diabetes progresses to the point of damaging organs of your body.

This does not mean you do not need any medication. You may still need your cholesterol lowering agents, your antihypertensives and diabetic medication, but you have to drop your weight to make a real difference. Let your doctor keep monitoring you and I assure you that he or she will have to reduce some of your medication when you have lost 10 per cent of your body weight.

Diet and heart disease prevention
You can lower your chances of getting heart disease by eating a healthy diet. For a healthy heart, eat:

+ less fat   + fewer calories
+ less sodium   + more fibre.

Eat less fat: Some saturated fats are more likely to cause heart disease. These fats are usually found in foods from animals, such as meat, milk, cheese and butter, and are also found in foods with palm and coconut oils. Eat less of these foods.

Eat less sodium: Eating less salt (sodum chloride) can help lower some people's blood pressure. This can help reduce the risk of heart disease. You need salt in your diet, but may eat too much of it. Much of the sodium you eat comes from salt added to your food at the table or that companies add to their foods. So, avoid adding salt to foods at the table.

Eat fewer calories: When you eat more calories than you need, you gain weight. Being overweight or obese is a significant heart disease risk factor.
Eat more fibre: Although the evidence is still inconclusive, eating fibre may help lower your chances of getting heart disease.

HIV/AIDS and nutrition
If you are HIV-positive, it is essential that you are informed about maintaining a healthy diet and nutrition. A preventive approach is important. Establish and maintain good nourishment early.

A positive, informed and focused attitude is important in keeping you healthy. Exercise is also very important. When you are 'up', the brain produces chemicals that help the immune system. A determined attitude is said to be characteristic of those who are healthiest. An HIV+ person must actively pursue routes that are known to help prolong life and raise the quality of life. Eating properly, exercising and taking supplements are excellent first steps! Just because you are HIV+ doesn't mean you can't have a good quality life.

While protein, fat and carbohydrate in your food provide building blocks and fuel for your body, vitamins and minerals are the necessary tools to enable your body to make the best possible use of those building blocks. Make sure you are not deficient in these supplements and they should help your body use the building blocks much more efficiently, and give better resilience if you get an infection.

While good foodstuffs contain vitamins and minerals, available data indicates that food alone does not supply enough in the presence of HIV, and that supplementation is very important (studies from Miami, Berkeley and Johns Hopkins universities).

Malnutrition may be a significant and early problem in HIV infection. In addition to malabsorption problems, nutrients such as zinc, selenium and vitamins B6, B12, E and folic acid are likely to be used faster than others. A good multivitamin should be considered. A minimum of 25 mg of vitamin B6, 50 mcg each of selenium and chromium, and no more than 10 000 i.u. of vitamin A could be a rule of thumb in choosing your multivitamin with minerals. It may help to take extra vitamins C and E and beta-carotene. There is no conclusive evidence though, that vitamins make a difference to HIV.

Nutrition and beauty

Diet plays an important role in maintaining the health of the skin. Your diet should supply all the nutrients needed to build health, namely protein, carbohydrates, fats, essential fatty acids and all the essential vitamins and minerals. Such a diet will consist of liberal quantities of seeds, nuts and grains, vegetables and fruits, supplemented by special protective foods like milk, vegetable oils, yogurt, honey and yeast. Nutrients play an important role in maintaining a healthy skin.

It is clear that vitamin B plays a pivotal role in maintaining a healthy skin. So a diet that is rich in vitamin B can go a long way in skin health. Vitamin B1 aids skin health by helping to keep the circulation normal. Vitamin B2 or riboflavin deficiency can lead to brown pigmentation or liver spots on the skin. These ugly spots usually disappear if generous amounts of vitamin B2 are given over a period of six months. Severe riboflavin deficiency can lead to oily skin and hair and small deposits of fat under the skin of the cheeks and forehead and behind the ears. More severe deficiency of riboflavin causes the skin under the nose and at the comers of the eyes and mouth to crack and become sore. Deficiency of many of B group vitamins – vitamin B6 or pyridoxine deficiency – can result in dermatitis or eczema. The symptoms may disappear when these vitamins are generously added to the diet.

Adequate amounts of protein and vitamin C are also important for skin health. There are many guides to antiageing diets. I am not convinced that you can really retard the passage of time (manifested on your face in wrinkles) by eating enough salmon!

But yes, it all helps and is therefore important to consume good fats in the form of omega-3 fatty acids (found in salmon and some nuts), and mono-unsaturates in avocados and olive oil. These oils will truly feed your skin from the inside.

Take action

One way to know if you are getting the Recommended Dietary Allowance (RDA) for all the nutrients you need is to follow the **food guide pyramid**. It provides from 1 600 to over 2 800 calories per day, depending on which foods and the number of servings you eat.

The assumption is made that if you choose a variety of foods from each of the five food groups (Grain, Vegetable, Fruit, Milk, Meat), then you will probably get close to 100 per cent of your RDA.

Drawbacks of the food pyramid

Much debate has taken place recently regarding the food pyramid and it has been modified extensively.

The major drawbacks of the food pyramid are that there seem to be too many carbs for the average woman. The fats are also all lumped into one category and women are advised to use them sparingly whereas research has demonstrated that you do need good quality fats. And if you are not on a calorie restricting diet, you can enjoy a good quantity of olive oil, avocados and nuts.

Traditional food pyramid

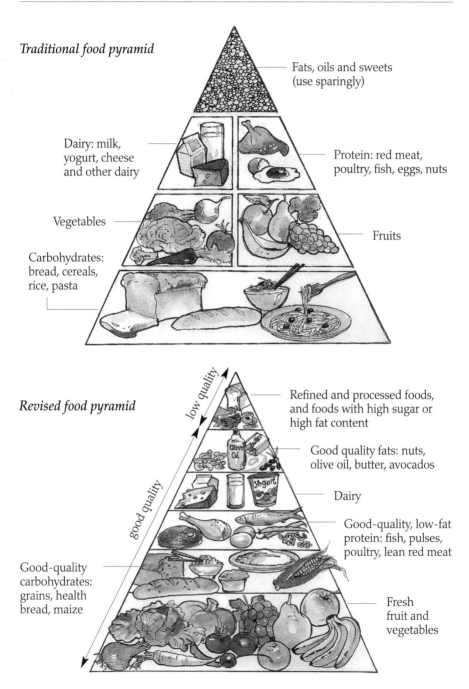

Fats, oils and sweets
(use sparingly)

Dairy: milk,
yogurt, cheese
and other dairy

Protein: red meat,
poultry, fish, eggs, nuts

Vegetables

Fruits

Carbohydrates:
bread, cereals,
rice, pasta

Revised food pyramid

low quality

good quality

Refined and processed foods,
and foods with high sugar or
high fat content

Good quality fats: nuts,
olive oil, butter, avocados

Dairy

Good-quality, low-fat
protein: fish, pulses,
poultry, lean red meat

Good-quality
carbohydrates:
grains, health
bread, maize

Fresh
fruit and
vegetables

145

Tips for disease prevention

☆ Eat a diet low in fat, especially animal fats and palm and coconut oils. (These foods contain saturated fat and cholesterol. Saturated fat and cholesterol can cause heart disease.)

☆ Choose a diet moderate in salt and sodium.

☆ Maintain or improve your weight.

☆ Eat plenty of fresh fruits and vegetables and a moderate amount of grains.

☆ Choose milk with 1 per cent fat or skimmed milk instead of whole milk.

☆ Eliminate fried foods and replace them with baked, steamed, boiled, broiled or microwaved foods.

☆ Cook with oils which are low in fat and saturated fat such as corn, safflower, sunflower, soybean, cottonseed, olive, canola, peanut and sesame oils. Stay away from oils and shortenings that are high in fat and saturated fat.

☆ Smoked, cured, salted and canned meat, poultry and fish are high in salt. Eat unsalted fresh or frozen meat, poultry and fish.

☆ Replace fatty cuts of meat with lean cuts of meat or low-fat meat alternatives.

☆ In recipes requiring one whole egg, try two egg whites as a lower fat alternative.

☆ Replace sour cream and mayonnaise with plain low-fat yogurt, low-fat cottage cheese, or low-fat sour cream and mayonnaise.

☆ Substitute hard and processed cheeses for low-fat, low-sodium cheeses.

☆ Use herbs and spices as seasoning for vegetables and potatoes instead of salt and butter.

☆ Replace salted crackers with unsalted or low-sodium whole-wheat crackers.

☆ Substitute canned soups, bouillons and dry soup mixes (which are high in salt) for sodium-reduced soups and bouillons.

☆ Replace white bread, white rice and cereals made with white flour with whole-wheat bread, long-grain rice, and whole-grain cereals.

☆ Substitute snacks high in salt and fat with low-fat, low-salt snacks. Chopped, fresh vegetables and fruits make a quick healthy snack.

Food labels

Reading food labels can help you eat less fat and sodium, fewer calories and more fibre. Look for certain words on food labels. They can help you choose foods that may help reduce your chances of getting heart disease. Words to look for:

✦ Fat-free

✦ Low-fat

✦ Low-sodium

✦ Lightly salted

+ Low saturated fat
+ Reduced or less fat
+ Reduced or less saturated fat
+ Cholesterol-free
+ Low cholesterol
+ Reduced or less cholesterol
+ Lean
+ Extra-lean
+ Sodium-free

+ Reduced or less sodium
+ Salt-free
+ Unsalted
+ Light
+ Calorie-free
+ Low calorie
+ Reduced or fewer calories
+ High fibre
+ More or added fibre

Read the food label

Look at the side or back of the package. Here you will find 'Nutrition Facts'. Look for these words:

+ Total fat
+ Saturated fat

+ Cholesterol
+ Sodium.

Look at the % Daily Value listed next to each term. If it is five per cent or less for fat, saturated fat, cholesterol, and sodium, the food is low in these nutrients. That's good! It means that the food in question fits in with a diet that is heart-healthy and may help reduce your chance of developing heart disease.

Practical Plan ✻

✻

Month 3:
TAKE ACTION
with food

Week 1:
Empower and
embrace

✻

FOR THE NEXT four weeks, focus on each one of these aspects. Maintain with Equilibrium, Excellence and Ease.

This is the beginning of a completely new programme. You are about to take charge of your body, your health and your life. This week you need to make sure you have checked out all your parameters. Are you up to date with medical checks: blood pressure, cholesterol etc. Chart your progress in your SELF journal.

Clear out your pantry and your fridge. Get rid of your margarine. Perhaps when doing your grocery shopping this week, you can substitute/add to it some low GI carbs – brown and basmati rice, whole-wheat pasta or sweet potatoes, as well as some pulses (chickpeas and lentils) to add to soups and stews. Choose fresh vegetables, herbs, salad ingredients and fruit.

Set your short-term and long-term goals in your journal. For example, A. (short term goal): 'In the next two weeks I will have started regular exercise and changed my eating style to match the SELF diet plan'. B (longer term goal): 'In the next three months I will have dropped two to three kilograms by following this responsible sustainable programme.'

This week you should also focus on appreciating the gift of your body. I know it is difficult as you stand in front of the mirror and are faced with those bulges or cellulite. Firstly, you are not alone, 99 per cent of women have some bulges and cellulite – it goes with the territory. Only ramp models and a handful of superathletes have a perfect body. Most importantly, do not allow self-loathing to creep in. Rather begin to embrace this body that has served you so well, that has perhaps carried children, is strong enough to get through the day of work, is fit enough to carry you through your life. Even if you have been ill or are suffering from a chronic illness, try and focus on all that is working well within your body. Your heart beats, your lungs breathe, your enzymes digest, your gut absorbs, your hormones secrete, and so on.

You must also begin to love your femininity. You are a woman and all women have something that is beautiful about them.

Come to terms with your body's limitations. This is a crucial step in the weight loss programme. Be realistic. The SELF diet ensures that your eating helps to maintain primarily your health as well as your beauty, your skin quality and antiageing and be the best you can be at each stage. Obviously if you are overweight, you have to eat less, cut calories and decrease your weight for your health as well as your beauty.

乆

Week 2: Exercise and eat
乆

Most diets recommend exercise as part of the programme while others may emphasise that most of the results (in the form of weight loss) are due to the dieting programme so exercise is optional. The SELF diet is different in that exercise is MANDATORY. This week you begin both – the diet and the exercise.

For the combination of *weight loss-health gain* you have to exercise! For health benefits (e.g. heart disease prevention, bone strength, etc), the minimum requirement is three times per week at least 30 minutes per session aerobic exercise.

For weight loss and body toning, you need to spend much more time engaged in aerobic exercise. You should ideally build up slowly to a total of five or more sessions per week for 45 minutes a time. The good news is that low-intensity, longer sessions are best.

You could swim, cycle, jog gently or best of all walk. You could do a combination of all (if, for example, you go to a gym).

This week find a partner or two and commit yourself to a walking (or other) schedule. Start slowly and gently for

10-15 minutes and each session build your time. Too fast, too soon is no good. Make the commitment and chart this in your SELF journal. Keep a log of each walk/session: length, duration, etc, and keep it going. This is the finest thing you can do to maintain good health and prevent all kinds of diseases and most importantly – you *will* begin to lose kilograms, centimetres and tone that body.

To maintain your weight and optimise health you must be consistent with your exercise, make excellent food choices and follow the principles and programme of this chapter. If you need to lose weight, you need to focus on three aspects:

1. Your calorie intake – what and how much you eat.
2. Your energy output – how much you exercise.
3. Your hormonal balance (i.e. the insulin story).

If what you are after is a prescriptive diet and you have patiently gone through this whole chapter and all you want is the diet – then here it is! Never allow yourself to feel deprived, even if you are on a diet. The SELF diet also means ENJOY your food.

Always consult your doctor before beginning a diet programme. If you have a very high cholesterol, heart disease, HIV or are on chemotherapy, I suggest you request a personalised programme from your family practitioner or physician.

The SELF diet is designed for a woman who is not pregnant and has no major medical problems but desires to lose weight.

Summary of SELF diet

+ Bulk of diet – fresh salads and vegetables
+ Moderate protein
+ Low GI carbs – attempt to restrict to 40-90 grams per day
+ Low to moderate fats – only best quality, ideally mono-unsaturated.

Breakfast
OPTION 1
2 scrambled/boiled eggs with tomato, peppers,
    mushrooms (optional)
1 thin slice rye toast /3 corn thins/2 rice cakes, tea and
    fat-free milk/herbal tea

OPTION 2
1 cup cooked oats with skimmed milk/fat-free/
    low-fat yoghurt
3 tablespoons low-fat cottage cheese
Tea or herbal tea

OPTION 3
half-cup cereal – All Bran/high-bulk bran/low GI muesli
1 fruit – orange/small mango/apple/half papino/sliced
    melon/ 2 pieces dried fruit – 1 tablespoon
Small serving fat-free yoghurt or cottage cheese

Note: The small serve of protein (e.g. cottage cheese or
yoghurt or egg) slows the entry of the carb into your bloodstream, keeping your insulin from peaking quickly and
thereby allowing slow glucose entry into your blood – and
the bonus is keeping you full for longer.

Lunch
OPTION 1
Very large delicious salad full of green leaves, tomato,
    herbs, peppers, possibly broccoli or spinach (made
    with love and creativity, when you have time)
WITH PROTEIN – half-tin of tuna or 2 boiled eggs, or strips
    of chicken or low-fat cottage/ricotta cheese. Add 1 (or
    maximum 2) teaspoons olive oil, lemon juice or
    balsamic vinegar, herbs and spicing.
You can choose to add a few raw almonds or a quarter of
    an avocado instead of the oil.

OPTION 2
Rye or whole-wheat bread sandwich filled with protein and salad (egg, tuna, chicken, sun-dried tomato, basil, rocket – make it interesting).

OPTION 3
Large bowl home-made minestrone or vegetable soup (make a huge pot over the weekend and freeze portions). Make it full of phytochemicals and antioxidants. (It is a good way to get your family to eat their supply of protective healing foods by adding soup greens, herbs, parsnips, carrots, a little pumpkin, baby marrows, broccoli, spinach, tomatoes, lentils etc.) Eat this with a sprinkling of mozzarella cheese or few tablespoons low-fat cottage cheese. (Leave out the bread with the soup – if you must, eat a whole-wheat/corn/rye cracker with it.)

Supper
OPTION 1
Huge delicious salad, different hot vegetables each night: gem squash, baby marrow, peppers , broccoli, spinach.
1 teaspoon olive oil with salad or few squares of avocado. Moderate portion of chicken (white or brown – without skin), baked/grilled or pan-fried fish (no batter – pan-coated with teaspoon olive oil), lean cut of red meat.

OPTION 2
Delicious vegetarian curry or stew made with assorted vegetables (as with soup, fill up the pot with nourishing, healing foods) and lentils and/or chickpeas. Season with cumin, coriander, curry leaves and Indian herbs and spices. Serve with brown rice or sweet potato.

OPTION 3
If you are eating out, enjoy grilled fresh salmon with vegetables, a grilled chicken dish with a delicious salad, sushi or a lovely vegetarian or legume dish.

Snacks

Enjoy a snack mid-morning and mid-afternoon.
Choose one of the following during the day:

+ a small fruit
+ a low-fat, low-carb yoghurt (fat count below 5 g, preferably below 2 g, carb count below 12 g per 100 ml)
+ a rice or corn or rye cracker (1-2) with thin peanut butter layer or fish paste and tomato or cottage cheese
+ few strips low-fat biltong (turkey biltong is best)
+ 10 raw almonds

At night, if you are the snacking sort, allow yourself a treat!

+ a small bowl of popcorn
+ 2 Marie biscuits
+ a piece of nougat
+ even 1-2 squares of chocolate (ONLY if you can stop after two squares, else don't start!)

In Weeks 1 and 2, limit fruits to two per day. Although fruits contain good sugar, on a weight reduction programme, cut back even on fruits to reduce your calorie intake.
As you progress, remember to:

+ be flexible
+ vary your choices
+ add delicious herbs and spices.
+ be creative with your cooking
+ love what you eat
+ use the best quality fresh foodstuffs you can afford.

Week 3: Energy

Energising foods

+ Food is energy. The fresher and closer to its natural state, the more energy is available from your food.
+ Make sure at least $^2/_3$ of your food intake is fresh, and include fruit, vegetables, pulses and grains.
+ Cut down highly processed tinned, smoked, frozen and convenience foods.
+ Cut down as much as possible on high-fat pies, pastries, deep-fried chips. Try and replace with healthy

153

alternatives such as pretzels, high-fibre muesli rusks/biscuits, dried fruit.

✦ Don't deprive yourself completely, especially if it brings you pleasure. Don't feel guilty! Enjoy a nice slice of cake occasionally. Replace high-fat snacks with boiled sweets or licorice.

This week is the ideal time to apply the 10 Healthy Diet Principles (see page 95).

⚹
Week 4:
Enrich
⚹

It is time to take a long hard, look at yourself, how you feel, why you feel the way you do and understand the concept of emotional eating. You eat for many reasons other than hunger. You may eat due to boredom or from frustration. You may eat when you are depressed, miserable or lonely. You may simply eat because food is in front of you.

This week, each time you are about to grab a snack, STOP and ask yourself a few questions (write them in your SELF journal):

✦ Am I hungry?
✦ Am I bored?
✦ Do I really want this?

And then answer (in your journal). If you are not hungry, tell yourself that as soon as you get hungry, you will either sit down to your meal or treat yourself to a healthy snack in a conscious way.

If you are bored, do something else – go for a walk, go to gym, turn on music, go into the garden and take a steaming cup of tea with you.

This programme focuses as much on HOW you eat as WHAT you eat. This week pay attention to these four aspects: mealtimes, eating atmosphere, pleasure and conscious eating.

1. Mealtimes

It is important to try to establish a pattern of regular meals. If this seems impossible, aim for at least one seated quiet meal per day. Ideally, the evening meal with the family would be best. If you are on your own this can be wonderful quiet time to cook yourself a special nourishing dish and to truly enjoy it.

2. Create the right atmosphere

Eat in a quiet and settled atmosphere. Don't eat when you are angry and irritable. Your state of agitation interferes with your digestion. Try to do something before your meal to relieve your frustration; go to gym, turn on beautiful music or have a soothing soak in the tub, and then sit down to eat.

3. Pleasure

Begin to truly take pleasure from and enjoy your food. Choose to eat what you love (obviously healthier choices) and take care in the preparation of your meals.

4. Conscious eating

+ Be conscious when you are eating or opening the fridge.
+ Do not just shovel down your food.
+ Be aware of what and how you eat.
+ Begin to eat food you really enjoy.
+ Eat at a moderate pace and eat till you are comfortable, not bloated.
+ Start to listen to your hunger signals. Start listening to your body!

CHAPTER 4

Exercise

Introduction

Beginning an exercise programme or improving your current exercise plan is the single most important element in maintaining your good health.

This chapter will provide you with a basis for implementing dynamic exercise into your life, and the fundamentals of exercise physiology will be reviewed. The remarkable benefits in preventing and managing chronic diseases will also be discussed.

Special topics are addressed, in particular: exercise and women's moods, hormones, sleep, sex, pregnancy, menopause, ageing and life stages. It will also review how to burn fat, how much exercise is enough for you and which types are the finest for women.

Physical Fitness: Quick Quiz

Are you out of shape, in good form or somewhere in between? Go through this questionnaire and then score yourself.

A. I exercise aerobically (continuous exercise producing sweat for a minimum of 30 minutes) at least .... times a week.

1 Less than twice   ....
2 Twice   ....
3 Three times   ....
4 Four times   ....
5 Five times   ....

B. How physically fit do you feel presently?
1 Unfit   ....
2 Below average   ....
3 Average   ....
4 Above average   ....
5 Very fit   ....

(Physical Fitness Quick Quiz *Continued overleaf*)

157

C. I am out of breath after walking up a flight of stairs/climbing a hill.
1 Almost always ....
2 Very frequently ....
3 Frequently ....
4 Occasionally ....
5 Almost never ....

D. I take a long time to recover after walking up a flight of stairs/climbing a hill.
1 Almost always ....
2 Very frequently ....
3 Frequently ....
4 Occasionally ....
5 Almost never ....

E. I have tense muscles and poor flexibility e.g. I cannot touch my toes with straight legs.
1 Extremely ....
2 Markedly ....
3 Moderately ....
4 Mildly ....
5 Not at all (i.e. good flexibility) ....

F. I have poor body and muscle tone
1 Extremely ....
2 Markedly ....
3 Moderately ....
4 Mildly ....
5 Not at all (i.e. good tone) ....

G. I am overweight.
1 Significantly ....
2 Notably ....
3 Moderately ....
4 Minimally ....
5 Not at all ....

H. My muscles are sore for quite a while after exercise.
1 Almost always ....
2 Very frequently ....
3 Frequently ....
4 Occasionally ....
5 Almost never ....

I. I am generally tired, lethargic and bored.
1 Almost always ....
2 Very frequently ....
3 Frequently ....
4 Occasionally ....
5 Almost never ....

J. I am generally positive about my body and its ability.
1 Almost never ....
2 Occasionally ....
3 Frequently ....
4 Very frequently ....
5 Almost always ....

Self-scoring:

Jot down your score results below, and calculate your percentage.

How many 1's ? Total = ... x 2 = ...

How many 2's? Total = ... x 4 = ...

How many 3's? Total = ... x 6 = ...

How many 4's? Total = ... x 8 = ...

How many 5's Total = ... x 10 = ...

GRAND TOTAL = ... %

What do your percentages mean?

90-100% Excellent
Keep up the great work. You are fit and in fantastic shape. Now you just need to maintain!

80-89% Very good
You have made exercise a priority in your life. You could do well by increasing some stretching and flexibility.

70-79% Average
If your health and fitness is worth attaining, try and prioritise some more of your time for your exercise, and stick to it.

60-69% Fair
Optimise your plan by increasing the frequency and duration of your exercise, and remember to include flexibility and strength training.

Less than 60% Poor
Plan to commit to very gentle training and you will begin to see results. Exercise is the most important fundamental in your health programme.

Sylvie's story

Sylvie's children were horrified when a group of researchers in the field of ageing suggested that she would be a good candidate for an exercise research project. The reason for their shock was that Sylvie, aged 87, was a resident in the frail care section of an old-age home. Her mobility was so limited that she was unable to walk to the bathroom without assistance.

The family were certain that any exercise would kill her. They finally agreed to a six-week trial in which she, together with 25 other frail care residents, would undergo a movement programme. This included gentle aerobic (cardiovascular) conditioning in the form of one-on-one training, and some weight-bearing exercises.

The results were astounding! The participants, aged between 85 and 95, demonstrated a marked improvement in coordination and balance.

These residents, who previously could not walk at all, had now begun to move around independently.

Note: This kind of research has been conducted at many medical centres around the world, all with astonishing results. A major centre for the study of human ageing is at Tufts University in Massachusettes, United States.

As a woman, at every age and stage of your life, the role that exercise can play in your health maintenance is remarkable. It does not matter whether you are young or old or overweight or even if you have a disability or illness, it is never too late to implement an exercise plan!

You certainly need to find a form of physical activity that you enjoy (or hate the least!). Try different modalities until you find the right 'fit'.

My story

My personal relationship with exercise only became serious about 11 years ago. Approximately 12 (relatively sedentary) years had elapsed since my participation in school sports. We were on holiday in the Cape with three small children and I thought that an exercise programme might address two of my concerns at that time.

The first concern was that I had been trying, unsuccessfully to shed excess weight in the two years since the birth of my twins. The second issue was my realisation of how little quality time I had spent with my husband in the years of our marriage. I decided that I would start jogging. I hoped that within a short period of time I would be fit enough to join him on his daily morning jog.

Neither of my two goals were achieved. I actually put on a bit of a weight initially (probably due to an increase in my appetite) and over years of jogging I never did get fit enough to join my husband on a run.

But I discovered that many aspects of my life and health changed. I was less irritable with the children, the quality of my sleep was enhanced, my mood lifted and my premenstrual symptoms (which I experience with intensity) lessened. The personal triumph was a fantastic source of satisfaction to me.

After about six years of deriving immense pleasure from my jogging as well as achieving a state of relative fitness, I experienced a set-back in my previously positive relationship with exercise. I developed a host of strange symptoms (see Chapter 1) and I was forced to stop exercising completely due to extreme fatigue, nausea, muscle pains and migraines that were markedly exacerbated every time I exerted myself.

Six months after a complete break, I decided to begin a different form of exercise. I chose something that was much less of a cardiovascular training modality and much more of a low-impact body conditioning in the form of strengthening and stretching. I began doing Pilates. It was a slow process of strengthening my central muscle groups (especially abdominal and lower back muscles), as well as building peripheral strength and good posture.

At first I really did miss the 'mental kick' that I had so taken for granted with jogging. But with the passage of time, the toning and strengthening of my body confirmed to me how much more women need than just 'cardio' (aerobic) training. In between I began swimming once or twice a week and then moved on to a programme of Pilates, stretching and yoga.

After many years without much aerobic exercise, I recently began a walking programme. I attempt to walk briskly three to five days a week for a lengthy duration with low to moderate intensity. That means that I walk at a slower pace than I ever ran, but spend much more time on the road. I also try to include a yoga class as well as Pilates or gyrotonics once each per week. This mix provides for me a combination of cardio-conditioning, stretching, strengthening and posture maintenance.

As I get older my priority in my exercise programme is far less on achieving the 'elusive great body' and far more on the maintenance of muscle and bone strength and a great, upright posture.

Design of the human body

Your body seems so solid – except for the voluntary muscles in your limbs, your bones and organs appear rigid – but the solidity of your body is an illusion. Just as the earth is constantly moving without you being aware of it, so too your body is trillions of molecules in perpetual motion. And the

161

best thing that you can do for your body in motion is to be as active as possible. The more you move, the more you enhance your personal health.

Unfortunately, due to high-tech communication and conveniences, the electronic age ensures that you move as little as possible. With the touch of a button you can open your garage door, enter your parking space, go up in an elevator and spend the rest of your day on a chair in front of your computer. If a message is needed down the passage or to your colleague in the next door office, you need not bother getting up from your seat, you simply send a quick e-mail. This ensures that you expend the least energy possible and barely need move a muscle other than your fingers. If you are required to ferry children to and from school, most of this can be done by dropping and fetching without much movement. When you do grocery shopping (if you haven't yet mastered it online), you are certain to circle the parking lot until you find the closest parking spot!

With all that has been gained in the e-age, much has been lost, not least of all the ability to move. In fact, the e-age is not particularly compatible with the design of the human body. *Your body needs to move in order to stay healthy.* If you think of any body function you will realise that it is all about motion. Consider the beating of your heart. This is a repeating cycle of contraction and expansion, facilitating the constant flow of blood through arteries and veins to every part of your body. Your breathing is a continuous motion of inspiration and expiration due to the ceaseless movement of chest muscles and nerves. Your food is digested due to persistent peristalsis (contractions of your gut). Even your thoughts depend on movement. Impulses must be relayed from nerve cells along nerve pathways. Your body is not a frozen structure. It is composed of trillions of molecules in constant motion. Your body is designed for mobility, not the sedentary lifestyle you may have addapted to.

What is fitness?
The word 'fit' is often loosely interchanged with the terms robust, able-bodied, in-shape or healthy. The strict definition of fitness really means conditioning and adaptability of your body. Physiological and biochemi-

cal transformations occur as you become fitter. Your muscle fibres strengthen, lengthen and enlarge. Your heart and breathing becomes efficient. At a cellular level, metabolic processes render you more robust and vigorous. Your body simply adapts and becomes stronger in response to the training.

The five components of physical fitness are:
1. Cardiovascular endurance
2. Muscle strength
3. Muscle endurance
4. Flexibility
5. Body composition.

1. Cardiovascular endurance
This is the most important component of your fitness. It refers to the ability of your heart, lungs and blood vessels to function optimally, both during exercise and at rest. Aerobic training, if done regularly and with proper intensity, will strengthen your respiratory muscles, increase breathing efficiency, stabilise or lower your blood pressure and improve your heart function and circulation.

2. Muscle strength
This refers to the ability of your muscles to exert force against resistance. You should have a balance of upper and lower body muscle strength.

3. Muscle endurance
Muscle endurance is highly correlated with muscle strength. It is the ability of a muscle group to sustain repeated contractions over time.

4. Flexibility
This is the ability to move a muscle through its full range of motions. It involves the interrelationships between muscles, ligaments, tendons and joints. Your exercise programme is incomplete if stretching and flexibility exercises are not included.

5. Body composition

Body composition is the relationship between your lean body mass (muscles, bones and connective tissues) and body fat. For optimal fitness, high levels of lean body mass and relatively low levels of body fat are desirable. This is usually measured either with calipers on several areas of skin fold thickness by your GP or gym trainer, or with a body fat measurement scale. The percentage of body fat recommended as optimal for women is less than 25 per cent. This is not always possible! My body fat just does not seem to drop below 27 per cent even at my fittest.

As much as fat is a taboo word, body fat is essential, especially for women. A level below 17 per cent is often associated with the ceasing of ovulation and menstrual periods. Women require a certain amount of body fat for the production of oestrogen.

There is no doubt that super-fit female athletes may have a fat percentage as low as 12 per cent but this is by no means 'healthy' in terms of female physiology and reproduction.

You can see that fitness is not a random concept but is based on scientific parameters. It is undeniably best for you to work on all five of these parameters, but cardiovascular endurance is the most important factor for your physical wellbeing and prevention of disease.

The physiology of exercise: how it works

Your body functions differently when it's at rest and when moving. Exercise simply pushes your system to adapt to the exertion or strain imposed upon it.

With exertion, there are specific changes within your body. The respiratory (breathing) and cardiovascular (heart and vessels) systems are challenged. The cardiac output (amount of blood ejected by the heart with each beat) increases. This is due in part to an increase in the heart rate or pulse (how fast the heart is beating). The respiratory rate (rate of breathing per minute) also increases. This allows for an increase in oxygen uptake needed particularly by the muscle cells.

As you become more and more fit, changes take place in your body which will be apparent, even at rest.

When comparing a fit woman with an unfit one, the parameters and physiological measurements are vastly different. In well-conditioned women, the heart rate will be lower and a measurement called the VO_2 max will be higher. This VO_2 max is the best overall measurement of physical fitness. It simply means the maximum oxygen capacity of the lungs. There is certainly a genetic component to this measurement in that someone like Bruce Fordyce (ultra-marathon champion) has a genetically superior VO_2 max. But sedentary individuals, by engaging in a programme of moderate exercise, can increase their VO_2 max by 30-40 per cent. The inevitable dropping off of this level with age will be much less in those women who exercise regularly.

Exercise is all about the working of your muscles. You have two different types: smooth muscle and skeletal muscle. Smooth muscle has nothing to do with exercise. It is the type found in the lining of your gut, the walls of blood vessels and within the structure of your uterus (womb). Smooth muscle is constantly contracting and relaxing. It is controlled by your nerves and hormones. The purpose of smooth muscle is to help the organs function. For example, the smooth muscle in your uterus is to enable expansion during pregnancy and contractions during labour and childbirth – all under the control of the hormones.

The skeletal muscle, on the other hand, allows you to move. These muscles are called 'skeletal' because they are attached to your skeleton. Skeletal muscle is under voluntary control. You can contract and relax any of your skeletal muscles. Skeletal muscle is composed of fibres. With increasing fitness and strength, the muscle fibres enlarge in size and also become metabolically more efficient. They are better able to use oxygen and energy molecules. The muscle cells function so well in energy production because they contain an abundance of mitochondria. Mitochondria can best be described as the 'power houses' or batteries of the cell. The muscle fibres are especially rich in these mitochondria.

For movement and muscle contraction to take place, oxygen is transported to the mitochondria. Energy is needed for muscle contraction. Fuel in the form of stored glucose provides the energy. As the exercise is prolonged, fat stores will start to be mobilised for an energy supply.

How to burn fat

There are many reasons why people begin an exercise programme. I would like to believe that the motive is to attain optimal health and prevent disease, but this is not usually the case. But it does not really matter whether your reasons for exercise are for personal power, well-toned muscles or sex appeal, the benefits to your health are tremendous.

The incentive in women, however, is almost always to burn fat! Although there is extensive established research in the field of exercise physiology and energy metabolism, the detail of this scientific knowledge is beyond the scope of this book. However, I will share with you the principles with regard to fat burning, the colloquial term for deriving energy from adipose (fat tissue) stores.

The secret is the **duration of movement**. As duration increases at any intensity, fat becomes an important fuel. You need to exercise longer and slower to burn fat stores. Interestingly, as your fitness increases, so does your ability to burn fat. So the fitter you are, the more fat you burn. It takes time to get there, so don't give up hope!

During exercise, energy is required to fuel your muscles. Your skeletal muscle contains only limited stores of high-energy compounds, called ATP (Adenosine Triphosphate) and CP (Creatine Phosphate). These muscle stores are only enough for a short while (e.g. a 100-metre jog) and therefore during exercise energy must be generated from other sources.

The three sources of fuel that generate energy to skeletal muscle are:
1. Blood glucose
2. Muscle glycogen (glycogen is the storage form of glucose)
3. Free fatty acids (FFAs) derived from general body (fat stores).

Energy is measured in calories or in kilojoules. In any weight reduction programme loss of weight is achieved with a calorie deficit (more calories are used up than are taken in). Even if you are sedentary, each day you need a basic amount of energy or calorie intake for brain and body metabolism in order to function. With a good exercise routine you begin utilising extra calories and thereby you set up an energy deficit.

There are insufficient energy stores immediately available to meet your extra demand, so your body generates extra energy from one or more of the above-mentioned fuel sources. If the energy supply is always from blood glucose and muscle and liver glycogen stores, you will seldom go into 'fat burning'.

If your exercise routine involves 20-30 minutes of fast and furious movement at gym on the treadmill, the bike or step machine, or a quick jog twice or three times a week, I am certain you have not achieved much fat burning.

The reason for this is quite scientific. There are three key factors in the physiology of exercise, in weight loss and utilising fat stores: the intensity of exercise (how hard you exercise), the frequency of your programme (how often you exercise) and the duration of your movement (how long the exercise lasts).

The first 30 minutes or more of an aerobic workout draws on your body's glycogen stores. The glycogen is broken down into a substance called pyruvate which then enters the cell's energy production cycle to create energy molecules. As the exercise continues beyond approximately 45 minutes, fat stores become important sources of fuel.

The intensity of exercise also determines the substrate utilised. Low intensity exercise preferentially uses free fatty acids (FFAs) first and muscle glycogen second. Substances released early in exercise, stimulate the enzyme lipase which breaks down fat particles (triglycerides) into glycerol and free fatty acids, which can then be used as a fuel.

The more frequent the exercise programme, the more likely you are to use fat as an energy fuel. From these principles, I suggest that your emphasis should be placed on *high frequency* (five to six days per week), *long duration* (45-60 minutes per session) and *low intensity* (about 60-70 per cent of maximum heart rate or MHR*) for maximising calorie expenditure from fat stores.

An easy way to remember this is by the 'FIT' principle:

F – Frequency of your sessions (at least three times, ideally four times a week)

I – Intensity (moderate intensity – build up a sweat, but breathe comfortably)

T – Time taken (30 minutes or more)

Note: With the load placed on the heart during exercise, the pulse (i.e. heart rate) increases. An average resting pulse rate is between 60-85 beats per minute.

For different exercise programmes you are advised to train at between 60-90 per cent of your MHR.

To calculate your MHR, subtract your age from 220. Then multiply it by the percentage. For example, for a 40-year-old woman:

MHR: 220-40 = 180 beats per minute

At 60 per cent of MHR: 180 multiply by 60 per cent = 108 beats per minute (bpm)

At 90 per cent of MHR: 180 multiply by 90 per cent = 162 beats per minute

Although the MHR covers a wide range, it is useful as a ballpark measure of how to determine the intensity of your exercise. A 40-year-old woman exercising at a heart rate of 108 bpm is training at a low intensity, whereas at 162 bpm is training at a very high intensity. If you choose to use this information while exercising, you can use a heart rate monitor or learn to take your own pulse intermittently.

How to exercise

A great body is desirable but has absolutely nothing to do with healthy exercise. You may be working out to improve your body shape (and that's okay) but the ultimate gain is to your bones, muscles, heart, immunity and metabolism. Unless you are limited by a physical disability or significant illness, you should be exercising regularly. If you have a disability or impediment in a specific area of your body, exercise other parts of your body if possible. If you suffer from an illness in which you experience fatigue and other symptoms, try a low-impact, low-intensity, gentle routine.

Although I have outlined some parameters for maximum benefits in working out, remember that any exercise is beneficial and just choosing to become more active in your daily grind is one of the most valuable lifestyle adjustments. Each time you walk that added distance to the car or climb those few extra stairs or potter around the garden, you are certainly burning a few kilojoules, working muscles and lubricating your joints.

After completing this chapter, it is hoped, you will feel inspired to take up the challenge and begin a programme of regular exercise. Please remember that most people, when motivated, dash into a programme expecting quick results which are impossible and unsustainable. Start gradually and train gently. You should not feel extremely breathless and pant uncomfortably during your exercise session. Take advice from nine times Comrades Marathon winner, Bruce Fordyce, when he advises that *'to become fit you need to exercise within your capacity, allowing your body to slowly and consistently adjust'. Too much, too soon, too fast will only lead to injuries and disappointment.*

Some important pointers: how to begin
+ Recognise exercise as a priority in your life.
+ Choose a form of exercise that you will enjoy (or that you will hate the least!).
+ Try out a few different options until you feel that it's for you.
+ If you can find a partner or group to join, it will double your chance of success.
+ Try to get your family behind you or even better, to join you.
+ Set yourself small achievable goals.
+ Start slowly.
+ Maintain . . . this is the greatest challenge.
+ Don't do too much. Excessive exercise is also bad for your health!

How do you keep it going?
This is the million dollar question. All beginnings are exciting and you may feel great after your first brisk walk or session at the gym. The second time you feel quite good, but by the third you may feel bored or utterly exhausted. That great enthusiasm in your first session helped generate an adrenalin kick which masked any pain or fatigue. But by the third or fourth session, you just feel downright uncomfortable.

After a few sessions, most people just give it up. Even with the knowledge of all the benefits of exercise, some part of you resists and dislikes the whole idea of it. You may tell yourself that you do not have time and don't need exercise in your life. Do not listen to this voice but rather take up the challenge to progress slowly, knowing that you have the ability to use a most powerful life-enhancing tool.

It is often extremely intimidating if you are an overweight woman to step into the gym and be confronted by ramp model look-alikes donning the latest designer sports gear! It intimidates you and me with our normal womanly bulges. On the road to health and fitness, you need to keep a clear perspective of your goals and your best possible outcomes. Do not set completely unrealistic goals. You may never have the figure to wear a bikini but you will certainly achieve your objectives of preventing or managing chronic lifestyle diseases, balancing your hormones, lifting your mood or relieving your depression. And if you still wish to wear that bikini, then go for it . . . but be the best and healthiest that you can!

How much is enough?
This depends on why you are exercising. To improve your health? To lose weight? To build muscle and strength? To perform sport at a competitive level? For each of these motives the amount of exercise required is different.

There is no doubt that too much is no good. You can overtrain and place too much strain on your body. You can also not allow enough time in between sessions for recovery of stiff muscles and joints.

The training for top level sports performance has become a science, the point of which is to achieve excellence. The focus in this book, however, is to achieve optimal health.

You do not have to exercise too hard. You never need feel completely out of breath and uncomfortable. Moderate is the buzzword. Ideally, to prevent disease, it is recommended that you work out at least three times a week for at least 30 minutes. If you can manage more, try increasing to five or six times a week and increase your time spent exercising. The key in all this is to train at moderate intensity. If you can increase your session to 45 minutes, five or six times a week, you will cut your risk of serious illness by more than 60 per cent. Frequent, lengthy sessions at moderate intensity will also help burn fat stores. Substitute low-impact flexibility, or stretching or yoga for some of your cardio sessions.

170

There is much to gain from building up a huge sweat on a fast jog, attending a spinning class or really pushing your comfort zone in your exercise. This kind of training is excellent as a stress buster or to lift your mood, and done regularly will create peak fitness. But bear in mind that if you are not a fitness freak or adrenalin junkie, moderate exercise is all you need for health benefits.

Unhealthy exercise

This seems like a contradiction. Isn't exercise and health one and the same? How can exercise be unhealthy? Your body requires activity and movement. But it also needs rest and repair. Yes, you can push further than your limit and go beyond your comfort zone at times, but do it too often and too much and you will land up with injuries and illness.

Overtraining

Overtraining is a concern in performance sports when someone is just not ready for the amount of training that is required for a big event such as a marathon. It is also an extremely common problem at the start of a programme. You are in a hurry to lose that weight or get slim and fit. But you cannot do it in a hurry.

It is difficult to give you a clear scientific indication of exactly how much is 'too much'. A few guidelines for health benefits include the following: one day a week is required to rest those working muscles. Training seven days a week is usually too much unless on your rest day you are doing a very gentle workout, such as a slow walk or gentle stretch. Spending hours and hours in the gym is certainly overkill. New research is revealing that excessive exercise stresses your immune system and damages your body. If you cannot get your training done in 45-60 minutes, you are probably messing around or doing too much.

But the common sense rule is that your 'body tells you'. If you are feeling unusually exhausted and you have trained the last few days in a row, your body is saying 'rest up'. If you wake up with a sore throat or cough, do not continue to train and pretend it is not there. If you have a new pain or ache anywhere (other than nicely stiff muscles the morning after), your body is telling you there is some strain. So take a break. But do not confuse this advice with chronic pain. Longstanding chronic pain from arthritis or back trouble does not mean you should not exercise. The current medical advice for chronic pain sufferers is to be as active as possible. The worst thing for your pain is to be immobile and sedentary. But please always consult your doctor before embarking on a new programme.

Exercise addiction

Exercise can become a most unhealthy addiction. Often some of those 'perfect specimens' you see and even envy in the gyms are victims of eating disorders, exercise bulimia and steroid abuse. Because exercise and fitness are so highly valued (and for very good reason), the fitness junkie or exercise bulimic goes unnoticed for a long time. They are praised and complimented and very few people, including family and loved ones, will realise that in fact the exercise has become pathological instead of healthy.

There are many reasons for exercise becoming an addiction. In many forms of exercise, the endorphin kick creates such a feeling of wellbeing that the individual cannot function a day without it, or she may even go back to the gym twice or three times a day. A woman with low self-esteem may find that excessive exercise helps create 'the perfect body'. This may give her the recognition she craves. Unfortunately, the effect of the recognition is short-lived which does not really make her feel better. Nothing can help her unless she begins to address the real issue, which is how she feels about herself. A few sessions of psychotherapy would be far healthier than the excessive exercise.

The person who has what is called an 'addictive personality' may use exercise (because it is so highly valued) to try and fill her emptiness. Exercise addiction becomes the excessive behaviour instead of an eating addiction, chain smoking, alcoholism, drug or sex addiction. It is more benign than drug addiction but there is usually an underlying problem that would best be addressed by a family practitioner or psychological counsellor.

A condition called exercise bulimia is well documented. This is common in women with eating disorders, who after a binge or even after eating normal meals need to keep working out to make sure that no excess calories accumulate. Instead of purging after each meal or binge, they simply exercise vigorously.

All these forms of exercise addiction must be taken seriously. Do not be fooled by the health promoting benefits. Exercise in excess is unhealthy and damaging and if it is rooted in a psychological problem, seek professional help.

Types of exercise

One day you open up a magazine article insisting that high-intensity training gives you the best body and the best boost! The next day a daily newspaper suggests that you have to do T'ai Chi in order to live longer and more healthily. Your best friend who has just returned from Europe says that Pilates is all the rage. Your colleague at work swears by yoga, especially for depression, whereas your ageing sister-in-law is training for the Comrades Marathon. Your beautician says she heard that walking increases wrinkles and you can get athlete's foot and thrush in the gym showers. With a whole lot of talk and very little action, you do not know who to believe.

An abundance of scientific fact exists, but there is also a flood of mis-information and myth. Do not believe anyone who tells you they have found the one and only approach. There is a great deal of value in differ-ent exercise modalities and especially in a combination. You need to take into account a whole host of factors in order to determine what is best for you. You are a unique woman at a specific stage in your life. You may be limited by an illness or medical condition or you may be stretched for time. You may not have the finance or the medical scheme that can help fund a gym membership or you may far prefer being outdoors on the open road anyway. The ideal programme includes a combination of car-diovascular training, as well as stretching and muscle conditioning.

Cardiovascular training

Cardiovascular endurance, commonly just called cardio, is addressed by the aerobic portion of an exercise programme. Aerobic exercise is defined as the ability to process and deliver enough oxygen to meet the needs of the tissues and cells during exercise. To qualify as an aerobic activity, the exercise must be continuous, rhythmical, use large muscle groups and be performed at an intensity that significantly increases cardiac output. Examples of aerobic exercise or cardio training include running, jogging, swimming, hiking, cycling and brisk walking.

Anaerobic exercise occurs when the muscle demands more oxygen than can be delivered in energy production. The muscle metabolism then becomes anaerobic which literally means it is happening 'without oxygen'. That means that energy is produced by a process called glycolysis and lactic acid accumulates. Certain sports with bursts of sprints include partly aerobic (*with oxygen*) and partly anaerobic exercise (*without oxygen*) such as rugby, soccer and particularly squash.

Walking

Whether you're just starting an exercise programme or are looking for something cheap and easy to do, walking is the answer. It can be done almost anywhere and is one of the finest forms of exercise. You will feel a lot safer on the roads with a partner or in a group. Remember to breathe deeply and walk tall, being aware of maintaining a good posture. This means holding shoulders upright and avoiding stooping as you walk. When you first begin your walking programme, start slowly, maybe trying a five-minute stroll. Keep increasing the duration with each session. Each time you walk, increase your intensity by walking faster and try to include a few hills. You can also emphasise arm movements. Because walking is generally a lower intensity exercise, try and build up to an hour per session, if possible.

Running

Running or jogging is a great workout. But getting started and staying motivated can be difficult. Before beginning a running programme, consult your doctor. If you have cardiac or orthopaedic problems or are more than 20 per cent overweight, you may want to try walking instead. Remember to keep your head level, your shoulders down and relaxed, and try and avoid stooping. You should start slowly for 5-10 minutes at first perhaps on a treadmill or a gentle flat road surface. You should build up to 20-30 minutes three times a week, being careful not to increase your mileage more than 10 per cent per week.

Swimming

Swimming is one of the best ways to get a total body workout. It has all the essentials – cardiovascular, strength and flexibility training all in one. The biggest advantage of swimming is that the water's buoyancy reduces your 'weight' by 90 per cent. Therefore your muscles, bones and joints have less stress put upon them. You can use equipment to intensify your workout. Use a kickboard to target your legs or hand paddles to target your arms.

Kickboxing

Kickboxing is becoming a very popular ways to exercise. Also known as cardio kickboxing and boxing aerobics, kickboxing comes in many forms. It provides a great cardiovascular workout and tones and strengthens muscles. Apparently the average person burns 350 to 450 calories during a 50-minute kickboxing class! Exercise at your own pace. Do not try to keep up with other people in your class.

Cycling

Cycling has become a very popular sport. It is a fantastic form of exercise. But take care to start slowly and build up gradually. And if you are on the road always remember to wear a helmet. Cycling gives a good cardio workout as well as muscle strengthening. If you are a member of a gym, stationary cycling is a fantastic way to do your cardio workout. While you cycle, chat to a friend, read a book, listen to music or even catch up on a TV programme.

Spinning

Spinning is a form of exercise performed on special spinning stationary bikes in a class within a gym or spinning centre. It is a high-intensity, huge 'sweat build-up' workout. You certainly get that adrenalin kick both from the power session and the disco music. This is generally not a beginner's exercise, unless you find a beginners' class. Please ask for assistance with the positioning of your bike and understanding the workout.

Dancing
If you like to dance, you can get a good aerobic workout from a dance session. You can dance in a health club, in a nightclub or at home. To dance at home, just move your body to some lively music! It helps to tone your muscles, improves flexibility and stimulates your cardio-respiratory function just like a good walk or jog.

Muscular conditioning
Over the years most of the attention for exercise has focused almost exclusively on the cardio component. This is probably due to the belief that cardiovascular fitness is the most important aspect for you. Strength and muscular endurance also form a very important part of any physical fitness programme. Good muscle and bone strength is necessary throughout your life for daily living, to prevent lower back problems and to help prevent the inevitable loss of muscle as you age.

It is unusual to spot a woman pumping away in the gym weight-lifting section among the bulging male muscles. Strangely enough, this kind of activity is even more important for women than men. For you to maintain good bone density and thereby prevent osteoporosis, you should be doing some resistance training. This means lifting a weight of some form. Obviously you do not want to pump up big muscles, so you would lift light weights or do circuit weights. You do not have to be in a gym to benefit your bones. You could simply do some home exercises with a 500 g tin of beans in each hand! (See the tips in the Practical Plan on page 191-197.)

Weight/Resistance training
If you decide to start a weight training programme, consult a trainer or someone to show you the correct way. Lifting weights improperly can cause serious injury. Be sure to warm up for 5-10 first.

176

Flexibility and stretching

The importance of stretching has finally received the attention it deserves. Flexibility is necessary to maintain an adequate range of motion for all your joints. Stretching should be done at least three times a week, ideally before and after each workout. It can be a part of the warm-up and cool-down phases of your cardio workout. Stretches should be performed slowly and progressively using a dynamic movement, followed by a static stretch held for 30-60 seconds.

The stretch should cause a feeling of tightness but no pain. Please do not begin to use stretching if you have any injury or medical problem or if you are over 40 and have done almost no exercise for a long time. Ideally, your stretching should be supervised initially and you should be guided by a trainer or attend a class of stretching or yoga.

Pilates

Pilates, pronounced Pi-laa-teez, is an 80-year-old method of physical conditioning. Numerous exercises are completed either on a mat or on various pieces of specialised equipment. This stimulating exercise technique is a wonderful means of conditioning and rehabilitation for people of all activity levels. Pilates teaches you that effective exercise is about quality rather than quantity, and that your body is an integrated system made up of interrelated parts. A large amount of strength is built up within your 'power house' region namely your abdominal muscles, lower back and buttocks. Pilates offers a refreshing change from more traditional types of exercise. You become stronger and more flexible without jarring or straining your body in the process. For those in rehabilitation, Pilates is outstanding. The Pilates exercises are restorative, safe and beneficial.

Yoga

Yoga originated in India four thousand years ago. Known most commonly as a series of poses which stretch the body, yoga is actually a set of guidelines for all parts of everyday life. Hatha yoga, which is the branch of yoga dealing with physical fitness, is the most popular. The practice is about a lot more than stretching (although it gives you a real good stretch!).

177

Most yoga practices involve specific breathing exercises known as prana-yama, which not only increase breathing capacity and strengthen abdominal muscles, but focus energy as well. Yoga often leads people to meditation. The word yoga means 'union' in Sanskrit, and ultimately the discipline is about achieving union by balancing of the body, mind and spirit.

The benefits of exercise

It seems almost too good to be true! Simply by exerting yourself and moving about you can transform nearly every part of your body and mind. There are marked physical, mental and emotional health gains. It is as simple as that: a dynamic lifestyle which includes exercise is the cornerstone of health maintenance. The difficult part is maintaining a long-term relationship and commitment to your activity schedule.

Exercise and hormones

Regular exercise has remarkable benefits for women, and the way in which it affects female hormones is important to understand. Frequent exercise has shown to increase as well as balance your circulating oestrogen levels. This is most significant in the transition through menopause or in post-menopausal women.

Menopause

In menopause the functioning of your ovaries declines. This means there will be a decreased production of the hormone oestrogen. Oestrogen deficiency manifests in much more than a falling off of your fertility. Among many other symptoms, it may result in emotional mood swings, irritability, depression and insomnia. It may lead to a decrease in skin elasticity, a reduced protection of your coronary and other vessels, a thinning of your bones and a drying and thinning of the lining of your vagina causing pain on intercourse.

The case for taking hormone replacement therapy (HRT) is strongly supported by the severe symptoms many women experience for many years. The subject of HRT is complex and controversial.

(Note: There has been huge media hype, causing a scare among many women especially in the past year, regarding the link between HRT and breast cancer. This follows the publishing of two very important global studies from the WHI (Women's Health Initiative) in the United States and the Million Women Study in the United Kingdom. Much of the reporting in the media was in fact inaccurate because the absolute risk of breast cancer with HRT was minimally increased.)

In all this debate and hype about oestrogen replacement, one point unfortunately never makes the headlines: *regular exercise elevates the level of circulating oestrogen in your blood.* What few people know is that oestrogen is not only produced in the ovaries, but also to a small degree in peripheral tissue such as adipose (fat). So after your ovaries cease functioning into menopause and beyond, there is still some production of oestrogen. What causes an increase in this production of oestrogen is regular exercise!

Regardless of whether you opt for standard HRT, alternative remedies or nothing at all, the point to remember is that exercise will increase your circulating levels of natural oestrogen. Women who exercise regularly have far fewer and less severe menopausal symptoms. Note that exercise does not replace the need for any hormone therapy, but rather serves as an effective enhancer of healthy functioning.

Premenstrual syndrome

Exercise also seems to balance the marked hormonal fluctuations that occur during your cycles. Disturbing symptoms that seem to appear for a few days, strangely recurring every month, are caused by those roller coaster hormones. Your menstrual cycle is affected by no less than four different female hormones: oestrogen, progesterone, luteinising hormone and follicle stimulating hormone. Each one of these hormones peaks and drops at different times during your cycle. Each one has a complex set of effects that keeps your fertility on the boil.

There are also many not so pleasant effects caused by these hormones peaking or dropping suddenly. Most significant is the Premenstrual Syndrome (PMS). The bad news is that PMS gets worse as you age. Each decade the symptoms may become more severe. And the more intensely you experience PMS, the greater the likelihood of a difficult menopause. The strategies to alleviate your symptoms include nutritional supplementation, optimising diet (see Chapter 5), meditation and medication. But a very powerful management modality for PMS is regular exercise (throughout the cycle, not just on the rough days). The exercise seems to stabilise the marked hormonal fluctuations, relieving many of the physical symptoms (including abdominal pain), as well as lifting mood and diffusing irritability. Some of these mood stabilising effects may be due to the release of endorphins and effects on serotonin metabolism (see Chapter 6).

Pregnancy

In pregnancy, it is essential to remain active. But always check with your doctor before embarking on a new programme, especially if you have any medical complications in the pregnancy.

If you have been exercising regularly before falling pregnant, there is no reason why you cannot continue your form of exercise until the pregnancy is well advanced and perhaps even to the end. As your pregnancy progresses and if you become uncomfortable, you can decrease the intensity and change the type of exercise. If you are only beginning to exercise when already pregnant, I advise that you join exercise classes specifically geared for pregnancy or that you choose to swim or walk gently. Avoid a very hot environment or extremely strenuous training as the marked rise in temperature may be harmful to the pregnancy.

The result of being active and working out in your pregnancy is great glowing health. Your hormones will fluctuate considerably during the different stages. The exercise helps ease mood swings, irritability, insomnia, nausea and discomfort. It helps keep your blood pressure at a good level, tones your muscles and ligaments and enhances your post-natal recovery both physically and emotionally.

Exercise and your pelvis

At a structural level, women who exercise have far fewer problems regarding vaginal and urinary tract problems throughout life, especially after childbirth and in later years. All exercise, especially yoga and Pilates, seem to strengthen the internal pelvic muscles. These are the muscles that play a role in bladder functioning and tone. There is always the possibility of developing uterine proplapse, bladder prolapse and some incontinence in women with advancing age and sometimes after childbirth. But there seems to be a much lower incidence in exercising women.

As you age and move beyond menopause, the lining of the vaginal wall will become much thinner and drier. Regular exercise certainly will lessen this problem (as will regular sex!).

Exercise and bone density

As a woman you need to take special care of your bones. From age 35 there is a natural decrease in bone density in all adults. This becomes more marked in women as you reach menopause.

Are you at risk for osteoporosis?
+ Are you a smoker?
+ Do you have a family history of osteoporosis?
+ Are you white skinned?
+ Are you light framed?
+ Do you not exercise?
  YES to most of these means you are at greater risk.

Oestrogen maintains the density of bones and as this decreases in menopause, so will bone density. To maintain strong bones throughout your life, make sure from a young age to ingest sufficient calcium-rich foodstuffs. Dairy is high in calcium but so are some plant products such as sesame seeds and walnuts. I would suggest that from your 30s you begin taking a good calcium supplement. Smoking exacerbates bone loss, so consider quitting for this as well as all the other reasons!

Most importantly (once again!) exercise has a strengthening effect on your bones. However, this time what you need is strength training. To maintain bone density you should do some kind of resistance training in the form of mild weight bearing. You could do this in a gym environment

Table 1: Exercise can do all this and more:

Ageing	Decreases your biological age and reverses physiological ageing changes.
Breathing	Stimulates and increases respiration.
Blood flow	The exertion, by increasing blood flow through the body, conditions your heart, arteries and respiratory system.
Cancer	Physical activity may reduce the incidence of some cancers.
Circulation	Stimulates circulation and thereby promotes cleansing of your blood and increased efficiency of all your organ function.
Cellular metabolism	Renders it more efficient.
Cholesterol	Bad cholesterol is reduced, improves your good cholesterol.
Depression and anxiety	May be relieved through biochemical changes.
Diabetes	Blood sugar control is improved due to improved sensitivity of insulin receptors.
Endorphins	(Natural morphine-like substances) are released engendering a wonderful feeling of wellbeing.
Energy	Is boosted.
Heart function	It conditions our hearts, arteries and respiratory systems.
High blood pressure	Hypertension is reduced/Improves your BP control.
Hormone and endocrine function	Is balanced easing premenstrual and menopausal symptoms.
Immune system	Is bolstered fighting off viruses and bacteria
Kilojoules (calories)	Are burned.
Muscle fibres	Strengthens, lengthens and enlarges.
Pain	Chronic pain may be relieved due to decreased sensitivity of pain receptors and endorphin release.
Risk	Reduces your risk of developing diabetes, heart attack and stroke.
Systems	Muscular, immune and nervous systems are strengthened.
Stress	Is relieved.
Sex	Is enhanced.
Weight loss	Is possible.
Zzzz	Sleep disorders are improved.

using the circuit equipment or free weights, or you could obtain some light (1 kg) weights and do some gentle exercises at home.

Exercise and beauty

We all know that exercise helps burn excess kilojoules and may bring us closer to our ideal body shape. But did you know that exercise actually enhances your beauty? Maintaining an exercise plan will improve your skin elasticity by raising your circulating oestrogen. It also helps oxygenate all your organs, including your skin. This helps plump up epidermal and dermal skin cells and helps shed dead skin cells. It may also enhance the detoxification enzymes in your body which neutralise and remove toxins. They are part of what causes ageing and skin damage.

Please remember, though, that if your exercise takes place outdoors (such as walking, jogging, cycling or outdoor swimming), always apply generous amounts of sunblock at least to your face, neck and hands. The sun is the greatest cause of accelerated ageing, especially to your skin.

Exercise and ageing

It seems as though you wake up one day and discover that you have suddenly become old. Wrinkles line your face, your hair has turned grey, your posture seems bent, your eyesight and hearing have deteriorated, and you just have to accept that body decay has set in. But this is not quite true. It hasn't just happened overnight and your body is not a frozen structure in a state of breakdown.

Beginning at age 30 (yes indeed!) and moving at a snail's pace, the inevitable process of ageing sets in. Changes begin to occur in your skin's elasticity, your hearing, eyesight, bone density, and muscle strength. Your metabolism slows down and physiological function declines. This is manifest in a rising blood pressure, inadequate sugar metabolism (leading to high blood glucose and diabetes) and increasing cholesterol. These changes occur extremely slowly and vary significantly from one person to the next. Some people age more slowly than others.

Today there is a worldwide interest in the idea of 'anti-ageing'. Much alternate and mainstream exploration is happening in this area. I am really not convinced that you can reverse ageing, but I certainly believe that *how* you age is to a large degree in your hands.

The three 'Ages of a Woman' are:

1. Your chronological age (how old you are by the calendar)
2. Your biological age (how your body markers and cellular structure reveal your ageing)
3. Your psychological age (how old you feel).

Only the first of these is fixed and is indeed the most unreliable. Two women at age 60 years may biologically be very different. One may have a biological age of 70 and the other of 40! No real regular medical tests are available to determine your biological age but in the area of scientific scrutiny, when cells are viewed under a microscope, the clogged deposits indicative of ageing cells do not appear equally and uniformly in all individuals. Some people have more advanced signs of ageing, not only in the wrinkles on their faces but in their cells and in their biomarkers (see below).

Many factors determine how you age, and there is no doubt that your genetics plays a role, but a host of other features contribute. A most important aspect is how you feel about yourself and your psychological age. How you look after yourself and manage your lifestyle factors: your nutrition, your stress management and exercise plays a major part in your ageing.

Below is a list of the 10 accepted markers of ageing. Evans and Rosenberg, exercise researchers and authors of the book entitled *Biomarkers*, coined this term to describe these physiological markers of ageing. They have demonstrated through extensive research that regular exercise can reverse all 10 of these markers. This is a remarkable breakthrough as it reveals that this process of deterioration is not inevitable. To a large degree, *you* can alter it.

Biomarkers

1. Blood pressure
2. Cholesterol level
3. Blood sugar control

6. Muscle capacity
7. Strength
8. Body fat composition

4. Body temperature regulation   9. Metabolic rate
5. Bone density   10. Aerobic capacity

Exercise and mood

You know that upbeat feeling that you experience after a good workout? It is probably the result of chemical changes occurring in your brain due to exercise. Numerous studies have shown that exercise *can* lift your spirits. There is now sound evidence that physical activity can also aid in treating clinical depression and depressed moods. Different types and intensities of activity have varying effects on individual moods. The studies reveal that after exercise, individuals with a depressed mood are more likely to report a reduction in anger, fatigue and tension as well as increased vigour.

If you are feeling really down and hopeless, it is indeed difficult to exert yourself. So take it slowly. You are also vulnerable to guilt and self-blame if you do not carry out the exercise. So introduce a feasible plan that is realistic and practical, not an additional burden. Try and find a pleasurable activity, and the best option is to work out in a group or with a friend.

Although much is said about high-intensity aerobic exercise, there is no evidence that any one kind of exercise has a greater impact on depression than any others. A positive outcome does not seem to depend on achieving significant physical fitness. Simply participating in physical activity shifts your mood.

How exercise alleviates depression remains unclear. It is thought to be a combination of factors. The role of endorphins in mood regulation has received considerable attention. These chemicals reduce pain and induce a feeling of wellbeing or euphoria. This certainly can alter your mood and leave you feeling great but it is questionable whether enough endorphins are produced by exercise to affect you if you are in a clinical depression. Another mechanism is that large muscle activity may help discharge feelings of pent-up frustration, anger and hopelessness. There is also ongoing research on the role of exercise in mopping up cytokines. These are inflammatory substances which aggravate depression.

Exercise is a most powerful mechanism for lifting and sustaining your positive mood. It is certainly a useful tool for preventing and easing depression symptoms when used as an adjunct to standard therapy, but does not replace the need for medication and psychotherapy.

Exercise and stress

Stress is generally experienced as a sense of being 'out of control'; exercise gives you a sense of control over your life. It truly is the best tension reliever. Regular exercise reduces the amount of adrenalin released by your body in response to stress.

With regular exercise your body becomes stronger, functions more efficiently and has greater endurance. You also now understand the effect of activity on your mind and mood and why regular exercisers have much less depression and anxiety. The balancing of your hormones, the increase in your serotonin and release of endorphins all come into play, generating an improved mood.

But exercise has another powerful effect. When you are exercising you do not worry! You are actually resting the nerve cells in the brain that worry, giving those cells time to renew themselves. (For further discussion on stress, see Chapter 5.)

Exercise and sleep

The beneficial effects of physical activity on sleep are significant. However, whether your exercise programme will enhance or even disturb your sleep patterns depends on the amount of the exercise, the intensity and most importantly on the time of the day.

Late afternoon and especially evening exercise has been shown to obstruct sleep patterns, especially if it is hard training and too close to bedtime. Possibly this is due to an increase in your metabolic rate which does not have time to return to its normal resting level. A low metabolic rate is associated with deep sleep.

Exercising at a moderate intensity for at least half an hour each morning, six or seven days a week produces the best effect. Stretching exercises also help you fall and stay deeply asleep.

Recent research from the renowned Fred Hutchinson Research Centre (Seattle, Washington) has shown remarkable sleep enhancement in post-menopausal women. With menopause, you are most likely to be struck by periods of disruptive insomnia and sleep disturbances.

The research revealed that only the women who exercised in the morning had the beneficial effects on sleep whereas those who exercised in the evening actually had more trouble falling asleep. One possible explanation for this is that activity affects the body's 24-hour circadian rhythm cycle. Morning exercise may get your body clock in alignment and balance.

Low or moderate intensity exercise for at least 30 minutes, performed early in the day, is what you need to deepen your sleep throughout your life stages but especially as you approach menopause and beyond.

Exercise and sex

For starters sex *is* a form of exercise! Lovemaking is good for fitness. A typical bout of lovemaking is probably equivalent to sprinting 220 metres. It is physically demanding on your body and every part of your body plays some active role in the sexual act.

Starting from the top of your head, sexual arousal sparks off the release of neurotransmitters (chemical messengers) in the brain which begin to stimulate the pituitary gland. This is the command centre for lovemaking. It triggers a cascade of hormones to regulate sexual activity. The pituitary also sends messages to the adrenal gland which starts to produce sex hormones and within seconds there is a release of adrenalin. This increases your heart rate, blood pressure and breathing. More blood is diverted to the genitals to prepare them for the forthcoming activity. Your blood pressure increases because your heart is pumping so much faster. The quick gasps of lovemaking indicate the level of exertion taking place in the lungs trying to rid the excess carbon dioxide from the rapid breathing. Muscle tension increases throughout your body. Your skin's electrical resistance increases to heighten sensitivity, particularly in the erogenous zones.

The gastric acid secretion is increased during lovemaking, possibly as a side effect of the adrenalin surge. This is responsible for the increase in appetite after sex. After orgasm (as in after the sprint) your muscle tension relaxes immediately, your heartbeat returns to normal and the pituitary switches off the cascade of hormones. The benefits and healing effects of sex then all come into play. But I do not think that you will get all your exercise requirements from lovemaking – unless you are a bedroom fitness freak!

The flip side of the coin is that exercise is most valuable for your sexual functioning. Regular exercise seems to balance your sex hormones throughout your years of turbulent cycles, premenstrual symptoms and especially menopause. Women who exercise regularly also seem to have a really healthy libido and maintain good vaginal elasticity and lubrication.

Exercise and specific diseases
Coronary heart disease
The concept that regular exercise (especially aerobic/cardio) will provide some protection against coronary heart disease is generally accepted today, although even supreme marathon running does not render you immune to heart disease. Other risk factors must also be addressed. But regular exercise, together with other risk-reducing behaviours (stopping smoking, healthy nutrition, etc), is believed to help protect against an initial heart attack (primary prevention) and in the recovery following a cardiac event (e.g. heart attack, bypass surgery) and help reduce a recurrent event (secondary prevention).

Hypertension
Regular training clearly reduces your risk of developing hypertension and decreases your blood pressure if you already have hypertension. A few studies of people with mild hypertension have found that half could discontinue their blood pressure medication after engaging in a regular exercise programme.

Cancer
A lack of physical exercise has been linked to colon cancer, breast cancer and lung cancer, with most of the research focusing on the link between

fitness and colon cancer. Please be aware that this does not mean that being sedentary will cause cancer. The research has just demonstrated a link. It is simply a motivation to become active.

Obesity

Physical inactivity may be one of the major contributors to obesity. In fact, childhood obesity seems to be associated more with inactivity than overeating and many obese adults begin their problem in childhood. Regular exercise is essential to deal with this problem. The emphasis of this programme is on long duration, low intensity and three to four times a week of exercise. Take it slowly and you are sure to benefit in all aspects of your health.

Diabetes

Exercise is positive for diabetes because it increases the sensitivity of the cells to insulin and thereby improves sugar metabolism. All medical treatment protocols for diabetes include regular exercise in the prescription! Check out your programme with your doctor as you will need to monitor your glucose more frequently and manage your medication carefully.

Lung disease

In people with mild to moderate asthma, a few months of controlled, gentle exercise can improve your fitness and lung function. Once again, please check out your medication requirements and details of exercise with your doctor. In mild obstructive lung disease you may certainly exercise (after consulting your doctor), but in severe lung diseases, such as advanced emphysema, it is not advisable unless under strict medical supervision and with extra oxygen.

Chronic pain

Today almost all pain management programmes include some type of aerobic and weight training programme. The good results may be due to a combination of endorphin release and decreased sensitivity of pain fibres during and after exercise.

Arthritis

With arthritis, slight pain may have to be tolerated during the exercise sessions in order to achieve the benefits. Your programme should work on increasing your muscle strength and range of motion but should not put excessive stress on arthritic joints.

Immunity

Recent attention has focused on the possible effects of exercise on immune function. Early research has shown that it may enhance the immunity. Frequent T'ai Chi, among other moderate exercise modalities, has been shown to increase the T-lymphocyte count. The research shows so far that moderate exercise may enhance immunity whereas intense exercise can have the opposite effect.

HIV/AIDS

A recent study by the Department of Health and Environmental Control in South Carolina showed that HIV-positive patients who exercised three to four times per week were less likely to develop AIDS than those who did no exercise at all. It not only slowed HIV progression, but increased blood counts as well. (**Note:** Please be aware that this is only one study, and this kind of research needs to be replicated.)

If you are living with HIV you need both resistance and aerobic exercise. Resistance exercise (weight training) adds density and bulk to the muscles in your body and enhances your stamina. It is very important to set realistic goals and consult your doctor.

If your joints are swollen, you are feeling dizzy, feel feverish, have open sores in your mouth or elsewhere, feel nauseous or have vomited, have diarrhoea, or have blood in your urine or stools, it is not a good idea to exercise.

If you suddenly feel excessively tired in the middle of a workout, do not continue exercising. If this continues, get to your doctor and discuss your exercise routine and possible adjustments to it. Exercise can also play a big role in controlling some of the side-effects of HIV.

Practical Plan 𝕩

𝕩
Month 4: Take action with exercise

Caution 𝕩

1. You are strongly advised to consult your medical doctor before commencing exercise if you have any disease, condition or disability which may cause you further harm as a result of exercise.
2. Please consult your doctor before exercising if you suffer from heart disease, diabetes or high blood pressure.
3. Consult a doctor before exercising if:
   + You have an illness or health problem.
   + You are pregnant.
   + You are over 35 and have not exercised for some time.
   + Your physical condition is poor.
   + You have injuries or problems in your muscles or bones.
   + You suffer from dizziness or fainting from minimal effort.
   + You are taking any medication.
   + You are unsure or suspect that exercise may be harmful to you.

𝕩
Rules on how to exercise 𝕩

1. Start gradually and train gently

Once you are motivated to start, it is extremely difficult to hold back and go slowly. You want the sweat build-up and you want the endorphin kick. You also want results. But for your exercise programme to be successful, this is the best way to get going. You want to be able to sustain it. Don't dash into it expecting results which are impossible. Take it gently and patiently. You ought never to get really breathless or pant uncomfortably.

2. Listen to your body

If you feel any unusual pain while exercising please stop and check it out. I am not talking about the nice pull of

191

unused muscles and ligaments. Rather, any unusual chest pain, sudden headache or a snap or spasm of an area of your body. Also, do not exercise when you are feeling ill, even a cold or sore throat can become dangerous with exercise. Rest up when your body feels excessively tired. Accept your body's limitations. But the usual lethargy and fatigue you feel in a regular day is no excuse to cancel your session. It is a very good reason to exercise.

Do not wait for energy to begin to exercise; the physical activity itself will generate energy. Try it and you will see!

3. Choose and explore
Experiment with different forms of exercise. Walking is a great start and a fantastic long-term plan, but add some strength training or stretching. Find out about what is available and affordable in your community. There are many creative and wonderful ways to bolster your energy, your body and your health, e.g. yoga, Pilates, kata boxing, aerobic classes, water aerobics, dance classes, mountain biking.

4. Find a partner or group
You will increase your chance of success with your exercise if you find a partner or even better a group to exercise with. The camaraderie of a group of walkers, runners or cyclists is special. You get to chat (which is a good distraction when it gets tough), you create warm bonds while experiencing the outdoors and there is usually a lot of laughter when the endorphins kick in.

5. Include the family
Try to get your family to join you or at least to support you. Set aside time on the weekends to tag along the prams, bikes, scooters or just let them tag along. You will be setting a great example, but more importantly it is up to you to create a healthy lifestyle for your entire family.

6. Find fun and pleasure

As strange as it seems, there is a pleasure element involved! The more fit you become the more pleasurable it is. It may be a challenge but try to make your exercise routine fun or at least less boring. If you are outdoors, change your route frequently to include interesting surroundings. If you are indoors, play great music or watch a good TV programme while you cycle.

7. You need discipline

No matter how keen you are when you first start or how much fun you try to make it, you will find many excuses to miss sessions or to give up the whole plan. You may even begin to dislike the whole idea. You need to make a head decision to begin an exercise programme and then stick to it. The essential qualities that you need are commitment and perseverance. Exercise is never a quick fix but a programme of lifelong dedication, a routine integrated into your lifestyle.

8. Remember to move forward

Exercise can teach you about your spiritual component; the need to discover, to take yourself slightly outside your comfort zone, to keep moving forward. You never stay completely still at any stage; you either move forward or slip back.

大

The Start

大

If you have been sedentary for years, you need to take your time to slowly rebuild your body. It is better to do too little than too much. You may be motivated to get back in shape and overexert yourself. When you wake up the next day with sore muscles and unaccustomed pain, you will simply give up. The concept 'no pain, no gain' is an absolute myth. You should feel fairly comfortable, especially in your aerobic training. Being able to talk to your partner while working out or walking suggests an appropriate level of activity, while breathlessness and inability to chat indicates excessive intensity.

Plan a schedule
Buy a journal specifically for this programme. Be practical and put it into your diary. The only way you will stick to your commitment is by planning ahead.

Set your goal
Be realistic. Take into account all your commitments and plan for a few weeks or months ahead. Write down your goal in your journal. It should not be impossible but should still be a challenge. Perform some basic screening parameters such as weight, body mass index and waist, hip and thigh measurements if you are on a weight loss programme. But do not get too hooked on these. Many of the fitness changes take place within the body as metabolism improves and muscle becomes more dense.

Journal your progress
In your SELF journal, keep an exercise record and log book! Keep a note of each exercise session: how much, how far, how long? And also chart down how you feel. Is it getting easier, unusually difficult?

✤

A. If you are just starting out

1. Week 1: The start

✤

Chart your success
You can measure your parameters, but most important is to notice your level of fitness, your mood, your sleep, your skin, your sense of personal triumph.

1.1 Find three 20-minute slots in your week and diarise them.

1.2. Walk for 10-15 minutes briskly at least three times this week.

Stretch: Do a 2-3 minute stretch following your walk. You stand still and slowly slide your hands down the front of your legs with your knees straight, dropping your hands as low as you can go. Then stretch a little further and hold the stretch for 30 seconds. Sit on a flat surface, back upright and your legs straight outstretched in front of you. Slowly extend your hands as close to your toes as possible. Try not to round your back. Hold the stretch for 30 seconds.

2. Week 2: Build up

2.1 Diarise three or four half-hourly slots for this week.
2.2 Increase your walk to 20-25 minutes per day.
2.3 Try to do four sessions this week.
2.4 Go briskly up a hill/steep road/incline to increase your heart rate and breathing.
2.5 Remember to stretch after each walk.

3. Week 3: Sustain

3.1 Diarise three to five slots for your exercise this week.
3.2 Increase to 30-40 minutes per session. Try increase your time spent even if it means decreasing your intensity. If you are in a gym, you can do a 20-minute walk and a 20-minute cycle or rowing.
3.3 Maintain! At least three times per week for 30-40 minutes. Remember to breathe comfortably through your exercise. If you feel dizzy or extremely uncomfortable, slow down. It is not good for your health.

You can substitute the walking slots with any other aerobic exercise such as swimming, jogging or cycling.

4. Week 4: Keep moving

4.1 After a few weeks of building up cardiovascular endurance, think about the other two dimensions i.e. stretching and strengthening.
4.2 If you are going to do some weight training for muscular conditioning, incorporate these tips:
+ *Warm up* Always do some cardio exercise first to warm up your muscles.
+ *Control the movement* Do not throw the weight. Lift a light weight for 2 seconds and then lower for four seconds.

✦ *Proper breathing* Do not hold your breath. Exhale as you lift the weight and inhale as you lower it.

5. Week 5: If you belong to a gym, try out different stretching modalities such as yoga or Pilates. If not, remember you do not need fancy equipment, you just need to stretch gently.

B. To retard ageing As for A. above, plus:

1. You must perform your cardio training at a low intensity, but longer duration and frequency i.e. walk slowly five to seven times per week for a period of 30-60 minutes.

2. Flexibility – Stretching is essential after every workout as well as a full stretch or yoga class once or twice a week .

3. Muscle conditioning – To maintain good strong bones you must do some weight training or otherwise resistance training.

C. To lose weight As for A. above, plus:

1. You cannot lose weight without watching your food intake. You need a healthy, wholesome nutrition programme that will facilitate a good energy supply for your exercise programme but at the same time allow you to shed those extra kilos (see Chapter 4).

2. To burn extra calories through your training you need to:

2.1 Increase your duration of your exercise. Even at a low intensity, you will burn calories if you spend much more time doing cardio exercise – ideally build up to an hour per session (but refer to section A: You must build up slowly!).

2.2 You should try to increase the intensity of your exercise session so that you push your heart rate up to 75 per cent of your MHR (Maximum Heart Rate) (refer to page 168).

🌿
*D. You are
already exercising
and want to
optimise your
health*
🌿

As for A. above, plus:

1. You must perform your cardio training at a low intensity, but longer duration and frequency i.e. walk slowly five to seven times per week for up to 45 minutes. You could change your type of training. Swimming is a fantastic choice as you would get muscle conditioning and flexibility training all in one workout.

2. Flexibility – Stretching is essential after every workout as well as a once or twice a week a full stretch or yoga class. A yoga session would add a new dimension to your programme as it balances body, mind, emotions and spirit.

3. Muscle conditioning – To maintain good strong bones you must do some weight training /resistance training. This will protect your bones from becoming osteoporotic.

🌿
Keep moving
🌿

Physical activity has the capacity to connect you, as a woman, with the functioning of your fabulous body. It brings you to an appreciation of your strength and ability. Use this to enhance your wellbeing and energy but always respect the power as well as the limitations of your body. Keep up your commitment and in addition to formal exercise there are many opportunities to be active throughout your day.

CHAPTER 5

Energise

Introduction

A lack of energy and the feeling of fatigue is an all-pervasive problem, especially for women. The term energy is derived from the Greek *energia*, literally meaning 'functioning' and 'activity'. All of life is composed of energy. Healthy functioning of the human body depends on multiple, complex energy pathways within your body, with continuous energy production and utilisation taking place. We can measure some of this energy through electrocardiograms (ECGs) of your heart, electroencephalograms (EEGs) of your brain and through magnetic resonance imaging (MRIs) of your entire body.

But energy is so much more than this physical function. The body broken down to its smallest unit is composed of trillions of atoms, in constant motion. These atoms are simply vibrations of energy that have taken on a physical form. Einstein said that matter (and the body) is nothing but energy in a specific form. Your body is literally a dynamic field of energy. So energy is in fact all three dimensions – structure and function and movement. From the perspective of quantum physics your thoughts, your emotions and you body are fundamentally the same. They are all vibrating energy.

Your energy level – *how you feel* – is a product of a large number of things but fatigue is most strongly influenced by psychological and emotional factors, the most significant of which is the experience of **stress**. Stress is simply how mental and emotional strain affects your physical body. So stress and energy are closely interconnected. Through this chapter you will begin to understand more about fatigue and learn methods to enhance your energy. You will also gain a deeper understanding of the stress response, what it does to your health and how to implement relaxation into your physiology.

Are you stressed? Answer the following questions and then score yourself:

Table 1: The Stress Quest

	Not at all	A little	Very much
✪ I often feel tired when I wake up			
✪ I often feel fatigued intermittently through the day			
✪ I find it difficult to concentrate			
✪ I worry about things that don't really matter			
✪ My stomach gets tense or crampy at times			
✪ I feel my heart racing at times (other than at the gym)			
✪ I can't keep worrisome thoughts out of my mind			
✪ Life sometimes seems just too demanding			
✪ I can become immobilised at times			
✪ I find I am indecisive at times			
✪ I feel jittery			
✪ I get irritable and frustrated with those around me			
✪ I pace up and down nervously			
✪ I sometimes feel overwhelmed			
✪ I am using more alcohol, cigarettes and tranquillisers			
✪ I don't sleep well			

	Not at all	A little	Very much
✶ I get neck- and backache at times			
✶ I feel on edge at times			
✶ I feel frustrated and on a short 'fuse'			
✶ I get headaches at times			
✶ I feel lacking in motivation sometimes			

Give yourself a 0 for Not at all, 1 point for A little and 2 points for Very much.

0-8 points: Although your scoring is low, it is still important to incorporate stress release and energising strategies into your life. Stress is a major factor in the development of all illnesses. Incorporate a technique into your life as a preventive, healing and energising measure. It allows your mind and body to regenerate and repair.

9-20 points: You need to begin to incorporate some stress busting and energy boosting techniques right away. People experience stress in different ways. Some women react to stress mostly in their bodies, while others have mainly mental responses. About half of women have both physical and mental symptoms. You have some features of strain to your mental psyche and your body, and you can achieve much more balance and energy with a few simple life adjustments.

21-42 points: Please be aware that you may be heading towards significant burnout and/or depression, and you really need to address your stress as a matter of high priority. Do not hesitate to consult with a counsellor or therapist. There is an area of overlap between stress, fatigue and depression, and there is much that can be done to assist you in achieving a state of functioning that will make you feel so much better, energised and at peace.

Nina's story

I first met Nina when she brought three children for a medical check-up with all kinds of winter coughs and colds. I remember thinking to myself that *'this woman seems to have it all'*. The family, the career and on top of it – gorgeous! I was aware of the successful business that she managed with branches in Johannesburg and Cape Town. She had just flown in from her fortnightly meeting in Cape Town – and home to sick kids.

At the age of 38, Nina had three young children and a highly success-ful business. Her day began at 6 a.m. with breakfast and the 'off-to-school rush', usually following a night of interrupted sleep. Her workday began at 7.30 most mornings and continued until at least five o'clock or often later. Lunch hour (if there were no meetings) allowed her to bolt out of the office to collect the children from school as this gave her a chance to see them during the day. She often attended to a few chores on the way back to her office.

Five-thirty or six in the evening meant a dash home straight into homework supervision and attending to family needs. Frequently office work needed to be completed in the evening and over the weekend. Despite all this she was extremely professional, always impeccably groomed and had a most engaging and warm manner. Even if there were opportunities to break this pattern for rest or recreation, Nina felt too guilty to pamper or indulge herself. Any spare time needed to be given to the family .

Each day was a fine balancing act, as it is for most women. For most women, however, 'carrying the load' is even more difficult than for Nina. Most women do not run a successful business, but work on a salary for an employer and may have more stress in meeting needs and taking orders than in making decisions and managing people.

A short while after this I saw Nina for her own medical complaints which had become chronic. She could not manage to walk into my office unaided. She experienced severe pain in almost every muscle from her neck to her feet and was extremely lethargic. After extensive investiga-tions and specialist opinions, Nina was diagnosed with fibromyalgia rheu-matica (a condition affecting joints, muscles and general body function).

Excruciating pain and incapacitating fatigue forced her to bed for a long while. It has taken many years for her condition to improve and for her to start mobilising and getting back to normal functioning. Now, several years later, she is much better but is still unable to get through a full day of work without feeling some pain or fatigue.

You may be wondering what Nina has to do with your story or mine. Well, Nina was a wonderful patient of mine and I couldn't help realising that in her I was seeing my own reflection. She was a powerful mirror which at the time I chose not to use. I convinced myself that I was attending to all my own health needs as well as dealing effectively with stress. Many years later I did have to confront the fact that I was indeed following a 'Nina pattern'.

My story

1996 was the watershed year for me. In May I gave birth five weeks early to my fourth child, a very sick baby indeed and I immediately closed my busy women's health clinic. I found myself in the same desperate situation that I had supported so many patients through: the situation of feeling emotionally and physically drained. *'All my inner resources have dried up'* is how one of my patients had described the feeling many years before I experienced it.

Although I had three young children and a very busy medical practice, I had up till now been doing all the 'right things'. I was eating healthily, meditating daily and participating in regular exercise. I convinced myself that I was maintaining a balance. I knew that the process of trying to live with energy and enthusiasm would be more of a challenge than ever before. After 14 months the baby's medical problems were well managed and under control. And I was on the way to re-establishing the elusive balance.

The situation became much more taxing after just a short while. I was surprised by an unplanned pregnancy. This not only gave new meaning to the idea of a large family, but was a huge mental and physical shock for me. I was in the midst of designing and delivering health and personal development programmes. I was not sure how I was going to cope with the strain of a pregnancy and an addition to the family. Fatigued and stretched to the limit, I tried to continue practising what I preached, but also began to try and incorporate new techniques such as guided imagery (which eventually resulted in my designing a series of guided imagery CDs for medical conditions).

To deal with the psychological and emotional stresses, I consulted a professional. Do not hesitate to call on professional help when the going gets tough – relieving psychological and emotional strain frees up your body and your energy. But shortly after the birth I was back into the swing of things – writing, lecturing, working, 'doing it all' – and then suddenly developed this peculiar liver and metabolic disorder (see Chapter 1, page 6).

This forced me to re-pattern my whole life. I was forced to rest much more. I became more vigilant with my diet and took good nutritional supplements. I began meditating at least twice a day and frequently used guided imagery. I temporarily stopped exercising and then changed my exercise modality to one of lower impact, more stretching and balance. But most importantly, I had to 'surrender' and change the tempo of my life. For me, the core of my disorder is about my energy pathways. It is about managing my stress and listening to my body's cues to maintain equilibrium and energy.

You are unique

The important lesson for me through this journey as a physician, a mother and a woman is that there is no one prescription to deal with stress or fatigue. You are unique and the task is to find exactly what works for you.

This may require trying different exercise modalities, eating pro-grammes and stress relief techniques until you find what is best for you. And then maintaining it through all your life's wobbly moments. When faced with new life challenges or traumas, it may mean digging deeper and trying a new approach until you once again feel in balance.

The problem with many life-enhancing or self-management pro-grammes is there is usually one plan to fit all. But your life has a specific rhythm. You have a schedule that is different from everyone else's. Your stress and fatigue triggers are unlike others and you may have a health concern or illness that needs improved treatment. It would be so easy for me to be prescriptive. But life and health are not mathematical equations. Life is continually changing and challenging, and one of the keys to dealing effectively with stress and fatigue is to have your personal health strategies in place. And then to be flexible enough to modify when necessary. This may be as simple as getting more rest!

As a woman in South Africa in the 21st century, you may, as I do, want to have it all: meaningful relationships, children, a successful career and good health. Isn't this impossible? And if it is at all possible, the question you may want to ask is *'Isn't fatigue and stress the inevitable price to pay?'*

I think not. Although perfect balance is elusive, attaining a dynamic state of balance is achievable. This is a balance that allows for falling, allows for moments of fatigue, and allows for imperfection and vulnerability. You can live with this balance by tuning into your own particular body rhythms, being flexible enough to stop when necessary, and most importantly by putting effective strategies in place for relieving your stress and enhancing your energy.

Fatigue and the TATT syndrome

Women of all ages and cultures seem to have one feature in common: feeling tired all the time. It is a widespread grumble that women bring to doctors.

Fatigue is defined as *'the absence of physical, intellectual and emotional energy'*, and chronic fatigue is a prolonged absence of this energy. For the overwhelming majority of people who complain of chronic fatigue, no specific physical cause can be found. But if you experience persistent deep fatigue lasting for several weeks, please go for a medical check-up. In a small number of cases, there may be a clear cause such as anaemia, a thyroid or blood pressure problem. Most illnesses from mild to serious will have fatigue as one of the presenting symptoms, so it is essential to get it checked out.

It is absolutely normal to suffer from episodes of acute fatigue from time to time. Acute means sudden onset and lasting for a short, limited period of time. This acute exhaustion is brought on by the demands of a specific situation. You certainly know the feeling of rushing to meet a deadline for work or sleep deprivation brought on by a sick child or newborn baby. This acute fatigue generally disappears with removal of the stress, the passage of time and some extra rest.

Chronic fatigue

Chronic fatigue means that this lack of energy is persistent, generally lasting longer than a month. You continue to feel tired, no matter how much rest you get. You often feel tired immediately upon waking and it may get progressively worse as the day goes by. Sleep is not sufficient to solve the problem of chronic fatigue.

'I am tired all the time!' were the opening words of 80 per cent of my consultations in clinical practice. I (tongue in cheek) called my practice the TATT (Tired All the Time) centre and my patients 'the TATT syndrome' sufferers, only to discover that I was not the first to coin this phrase. 'Tired all the time' is a universal malady. In the overwhelming majority of cases no physical cause can be found. In describing the TATT syndrome I am not referring to a condition called the Chronic Fatigue Syndrome.

Chronic Fatigue Syndrome (CFS)

Chronic Fatigue Syndrome is a condition also known as M.E. (myalgic encephalomyelitis), yuppie flu, post-viral fatigue syndrome, Royal Free Hospital disease or chronic Epstein-Barr virus syndrome. CFS is a newly established syndrome that describes varying combinations of symptoms, including recurrent fatigue, sore throats, low grade fever, muscle and joint pain, recurrent headache and loss of concentration, among others. Although newly defined, currently popular and still somewhat controversial within the medical profession, CFS is not a new disease at all. References to a similar condition in medical literature go back as far as the 1860s.

CFS is not taken seriously by many doctors and most medically trained allopathic doctors do not believe it is a real condition at all. In 1988 it was formally defined by a consensus panel convened by the Centre of Disease Control (CDC) in Atlanta. A formal set of criteria was established by the CDC and then followed by British and Australian criteria.

Researchers who focused on identifying an infectious agent as the cause of CFS found the Epstein-Barr virus the leading, yet controversial candidate. Other viruses from the herpes group have also been identified, including herpes type 1 and 2, varicella zoster virus and cytomegalovirus. These viruses have an ability to establish a lifelong latent infection after the initial infection.

There are, however, many other causes other than infectious agents. Environmental illness, impaired liver function, excessive gastrointestinal permeability, chronic candida infection and food allergies have been listed. A disturbed immune system usually plays a central role in this condition. It is a very difficult condition to manage, often compounded by the fact that your doctor may not believe it is real or have very little experience in managing the syndrome. You may have to search to find a compassionate and skilled physician to help you through this. It is always important to find any underlying health problems.

The most effective treatment is a comprehensive lifestyle programme that is designed to help fuel higher energy levels with nutrition, exercise, supplements, stress management and avoidance of precipitants.

Energy
At any given moment your energy level is a product of a large number of things: the quality of the food you eat, your digestion, your level of activity, the quality of your sleep, the temperature of the air around you, and your thoughts and emotions. To live with greater energy means addressing all aspects of your lifestyle. Exercise (Chapter 4), energising food choices and good digestion (Chapter 3) and emotional wellbeing (Chapter 2) are all essential components to combat fatigue and live with greater energy.

Notwithstanding all the important factors already mentioned, it has become clear that most chronic fatigue is strongly influenced by emotional and psychological factors, the most significant of which is the experience of stress.

The mind-emotions-body connection

Every time you think a thought or feel an emotion, a chemical messenger is produced. The name for these chemicals are neuropeptides (or nerve proteins). An example of how these messengers work is expressed in your immune function. For example, when your thoughts are angry, critical and resentful, a chemical messenger is produced which depresses your immune system. When your thoughts are loving and empowering, the nerve protein messenger actually enhances your immune function. Research into these pathways demonstrate that antibody activity is increased, T-cell lymphocytes and Natural Killer (NK) cells (a type of immune cell) are stimulated when you produce positive thoughts and images.

Constant communication takes place between our brain and body systems through these nerve proteins. They have a powerful effect on all processes in your body, including energy production. A deficit in your emotional life and stress to your mental state literally robs your body of energy and produces fatigue. This energy drain is a function of the mind-body connection.

The ability of a patient's mind to affect the process of virtually every disease has been well documented. The body of knowledge in scientific literature documenting the critical importance of a patient's psyche on the therapeutic environment has grown tremendously. A major study published in the illustrious journal *Lancet* in September 2004 revealed across 52 countries that in the year prior to their heart attack, patients had been under significantly more stress – from work, family, financial troubles, depression and other causes in the vast majority of cases. Dr Salim Yusuf of McMaster University says that stress is as great a risk factor for heart disease as hypertension and obesity.

An interesting area of study is on how the substances called endorphins function. Endorphins are naturally produced 'morphine-like' substances. They are released from central (brain) and peripheral (nerve) areas of the body in response to pain, stress and emotions and perform many functions of which analgesia (pain relief) is but one. They, too, enhance the function of the immune system. It is becoming evident that

208

the boundaries between the central nervous system and the immune system are not as clear as once thought.

The experience of stress is a clear manifestation of the mind-emotion-body pathway. Mental or emotional strain causes the direct production and release of adrenalin within your body which in turn affects many different physical functions. So a thought or emotion sets off a cascade of events, resulting in physical body changes.

Stress response

Any disturbance in your body, such as physical trauma, a danger, a strong emotional reaction (anger), crossing a busy street or a presentation, may trigger what is called 'the stress response'. You may or may not be conscious of the response happening in your body, and it is a major factor in producing fatigue.

Life equals stress. You can no more eliminate stress from your life than you can eliminate tension from your muscles. If muscle tension dropped to nothing, you would fall to the ground in a shapeless heap. So, too, if all stress disappeared, you would not function. It's only when it becomes overwhelming that it becomes problematic. You need some 'good stress' or 'challenge' in order to thrive and move through life with the passion and purpose required for energised living.

Unfortunately, most of your life circumstances push you into overwhelming, simmering stress. And it's this negative stress that causes all the harm. Your daily stresses have become so much a part of your life that you have resigned yourself to the reality of getting on with it and 'coping' with them. Stress is unfortunately highly valued in the workplace. Extended overtime work schedules and unrelenting slog is often praised. Even women who are not in the workplace continually moan and even compete with each other about how busy, how stressed and how 'hectic' life is.

The result of this simmering stress is an infiltration into your mental psyche, a depletion of your emotional resources and a corrosion of the cells of your body. You literally get sick at all levels. It may be a slow process or a sudden event. For some people it manifests in life-threatening conditions, while for the majority of people it may transform into frequent nagging headaches, back pain or an irritable colon. No-one escapes the inevitable havoc played out by stress within the body. In many individuals it may result in a catastrophic heart attack. The Japanese have a word for it: *Karoshi* – death by overwork.

You have to face stressful events each and every day with which you can usually cope. It is when the stressful situation becomes unrelenting that damage begins to occur. As your worries envelop you in a black cloud, there is an outpouring of stress hormones which wear out the adrenal gland and deplete your immune system. The most extreme result is the condition commonly known as 'burnout'.

What causes stress?
Stress is a simple way to explain how mental strain affects your physical body. At it simplest, stress is the release of adrenalin in your body.

Mounting bills, unreasonable work demands, difficult children or the threat of crime keep you from feeling at ease. It is easy to think that the external stressors are the cause of your tension. But it's how you respond to them that causes the stress.

Unfortunately, you are powerless to change many of these life factors. You can, however, tackle your *internal* responses to these stressors. Your reactions to these 'obstacles of living' manifest in anxiety, fearfulness and depression. This internalised stress keeps your mind agitated, interferes with your immune system and produces stress-related ailments. But you can learn to change your reactions to the stresses of life (see page 215).

Specific body (physiological) changes occur in stressful situations. These changes are called the *fight-flight reaction*. The primitive response of your body to stress is either to flee or to fight. Have you ever thought *'Why does my heart beat faster or my palms get sweaty or my muscles tense up when I have to do a presentation?'* The fight-flight reaction is the body's physical response to danger.

As soon as a message of 'Danger' is picked up by the brain, it then transfers this signal through the nervous system. As soon as your body experiences a danger or perceived danger (stress), it starts to mobilise 'its forces' for immediate activity. The sudden onset of palpitations, a thumping heart, sweaty palms, shallow quick breathing and tense muscles occur. The hormones adrenaline and cortisol are released from your body. Your heart begins to race in order to increase it's output, thereby raising blood pressure. Blood is shunted away from your central digestive organs, rushing to your muscles and brain. Your muscles tense up in anticipation of a fight or a sprint. Breathing is quickened and shallow. The pupils of your eyes dilate, facilitating acute vision. Stomach acids flow, helping to mobilise as much sugar as possible. This increased glucose is needed for for brain usage.

The amazing thing is that your body responds in an identical manner whether you are actually in danger, for example, within a burning building or facing an attack, or just thinking about it!

This is all very helpful if indeed you are escaping burning buildings or fighting off wild bears. But unfortunately your body responds in the same way in traffic jams, board meetings and throughout the course of a regular day. The cascade of stress hormones is triggered and you neither fight nor flee. Instead the stress simmers away inside you. You may have adapted to such chronically high levels of stress that you now assume this state to be normal.

You may be so tangled up in stress that you are not even aware of this sustained fight-flight going on inside you. Even when you are sleeping, you may thrash about, grind your teeth and wake up unrefreshed in the morning.

The general adaptation syndrome

The stress response is actually part of a larger response called the 'general adaptation syndrome'. This syndrome is composed of three phases, which are controlled and regulated by the adrenal glands.

1. Phase I = ALARM reaction. The alarm reaction is generally the fight-flight response described above. It is designed to counteract danger by mobilising your body's resources for immediate physical activity. It is mainly due to the release of adrenalin.
2. Phase II = RESISTANCE reaction. While the alarm phase is usually short-lived, the next phase, the resistance reaction, allows your body

to continue fighting long after the effects of the fight-flight reaction have worn off. Other hormones, such as cortisol, are mobilised and are largely responsible for the resistance reaction. For example, these hormones make sure the body has a large supply of energy long after the glucose has been used. They also promote the retention of sodium to keep your blood pressure elevated. Prolongation of the resistance reaction places further strain on body and increases the risk of illness and damage.

3. Phase III = EXHAUSTION reaction. Prolonged stress places a tremendous load on many organ systems, especially the heart, blood vessels, adrenals and the immune system. It may present as a partial or total collapse of a body function.

The paradox

The release of adrenalin (or fight-flight) is an amazing body function designed to **protect** your body from danger. It is designed to counteract danger by mobilising your body's resources for immediate action.

The paradox of this stress response is that although it is designed to counteract danger and therefore minimise damage, it effectively lands up causing damage! The reason for this is that most of the time that this system is firing away is not in response to a life threat but to that of the daily strain of life.

Possible long-term effects linked to stress:

+ Allergies
+ Depression, Anxiety, Insomnia
+ 'Burnout'
+ Stomach ulcers

+ Arthritis
+ Headaches
+ Hypertension
+ Immune supression

What should you do about it?

Whether you are aware of it or not, you have developed a pattern for coping with stress. Unfortunately, most coping patterns/methods do not support good health. Negative coping patterns include smoking more, consuming more alcohol, overeating, switching off from the world and retreating into television, emotional outbursts or inappropriate anger and overspending.

Managing stress

The critical factor between stress being harmful or not is based on the strength of your whole body system. Managing your stress can be divided into five sections:

1. Lifestyle factors
2. Exercise
3. Nourishing diet to support physiological processes (biochemistry)
4. Supplements
5. Techniques to calm your mind and thereby trigger the relaxation response

The key to managing stress is understanding a physiological body state called the relaxation response. The exact opposite of what happens to your body during stress is what occurs in the relaxation response. Sounds simple? All you need to do is turn on the TV, put up your feet and relax? No! It does not happen automatically.

Your body and your mind no longer know how to switch from one system to another automatically. From stress response to relaxation response, from sympathetic to parasympathetic nervous system function. You need to teach your mind and body techniques to produce this parasympathetic relaxation response.

Stress managing factors

1. Your *lifestyle* is the main determinant in your stress levels. It is not necessarily the workload that is the main culprit. Research demonstrates that the two most potent stressors are lack of time management and relationship problems at home and at work!
2. As simple and common sense as it seems, exercise is a powerful stress buster. With regular exercise your body becomes stronger, functions more efficiently and has greater endurance. Regular exercisers have much less depression and are less likely to suffer from fatigue or anxiety. Exercise alone (with nothing else) has been

213

shown to have a dramatic impact on improving mood and ability to handle stressful life situations.

3. With stress you also need to support the *biochemistry* of your body:
   + Cut caffeine
   + Restrict alcohol (alcohol produces a chemical stress on the body and increases adrenalin output and interferes with brain chemistry)
   + Cut refined carbohydrates (rather eat low GI carbs), sugar and flour
   + Eat more whole foods (with antioxidants)
   + Increase minerals especially K (potassium) and Mg (magnesium).

4. *Supplements:* Vitamins C, B6, zinc and magnesium all play a critical role in the health of the adrenal gland. During stress these levels decrease significantly. Therefore delivery of high quality nutrition to the cells of your body is a critical factor in determining your resilience.

5. *The Relaxation Response:* You have the power to create internal harmony instead of internal tension. The introduction of potent stress management skills into your life provides your body with the physiological experience to fight off stress. It allows your mind and body time to repair, regenerate and recover from the wear and tear of everyday strain.

When you engage in a sound relaxation technique you simply shift your body to a state in which it functions in the opposite way to fight-flight. Your heart rate will slow and blood pressure will drop. Your breathing deepens and your entire body is oxygenated. Your muscles relax and your blood is shunted back to the central organs aiding digestion and metabolism. Your blood sugar as well as stomach acid returns to normal levels.

All this is what happens to you on a physical level. The emotional and psychological effects are even more profound. Your mood is shifted into a more joyous state, and with regular relaxation exercises, your depression and anxiety may be relieved. While the sympathetic nervous system is designed to protect your body from immediate danger, the parasympathetic system is designed for repair, maintenance and restoration of the body.

The good news is that you do not need much time for your body to be in this state: a minimum of 10-20 minutes or short five-minute power breaks during the day.

The science of cycles

Everything moves and flows in cycles. You can see this cyclical nature in day and night, high and low tides, and seasonal changes. The cycles of contraction and expansion are apparent in your pulse and heartbeat, your breathing, digestion, muscle function and the cycles of cell and tissue regeneration.

As night moves into day, your vital body functions, including heart rate and blood pressure, speed up in anticipation of increased physical activity. Every aspect of life is cyclical.

Chronobiology is the name given to this relatively new science. Chronobiology studies what ancient wisdoms recognised thousands of years ago: that everything operates in cycles. It identifies the physiology of the rhythms that control and influence your functioning. A simple understanding of this may enable you to live with increased energy, balance and harmony.

Within your body are many different biological clocks located in your brain, each regulating important processes according to specific time cycles. The most important of these is called the circadian rhythm. It is a 24-hour cycle. This clock is very important as so many of your normal bodily functions follow a daily pattern of speeding up and slowing down in tune with this clock. This internal 'clock' controls your hormones, chemicals, nervous function and sleep-wake cycles. Although these biorhythms can be reprogrammed by environmental influences (such as night work), they are genetically 'hard-wired' into your cells, tissue and organs.

The following examples demonstrate how this internal clock (circadian rhythm) functions in your body. There are times in the day optimum for digestion, periods for improved concentration and good phases for creative thought.

215

✦ Your body temperature increases throughout the day, reaching a high point in the late afternoon, then decreases to its lowest point after midnight.

✦ The production of the anti-stress hormone cortisol is somewhat different. It peaks predictably at around seven in the morning, and reaches its low point in the evening.

✦ Digestion is much less efficient later at night than at midday. The middle of the day is when your digestion is at its peak and it is a good idea to have your large meal then.

✦ Mid-morning seems to be the time of day when your concentration and creative thought is at its peak.

These simple pieces of information encourage you to take heed of the concept 'pace yourself'. Utilising this knowledge could dramatically enhance each day. For example, schedule your most challenging meetings or work projects for earlier in the morning when the anti-stress hormone is most functional.

By understanding this information you realise that a human being is not designed to function in a relentless, sustained fashion (even the human woman!). That is not how the universe functions. There is time for activity and time for rest. Contraction and expansion implies a building up and then a gearing down. A muscle in a continuous expanded state would simply snap. The heart muscle in particular would collapse.

How can you expect to live with health and achieve balance when you continue to drive yourselves at the high-speed pace of the 21st century towards possible illness and burnout?

Burnout

Burnout is not actually a medical diagnosis. It is a colloquial term that has found its way into health dictionaries, but it is nevertheless a real experience. It describes a state of extreme stress, where you can reach a point of becoming ill and often non-functional. Burnout is defined as a state of mental and/or physical exhaustion caused by excessive and prolonged stress. The experience of stress can be compared to an elastic band. With continuous stress, the band is stretched and stretched but keeps bouncing back, often not to its original state but it does resume some shape. With burnout, the elastic snaps – there is no bouncing back. The process progresses through stages, giving you the opportunity to recognise symptoms and take preventive steps. The exhaustion stage is where most people realise that something is wrong. Symptoms include depression, stomach or bowel problems, mental fatigue, chronic headaches or migraines, anger, the desire to 'drop out' of society or to get away from it all.

What causes burnout?
+ Unrelenting stress
+ Trying to be all things to all people
+ Trying to meet everyone's demands and expectations
+ Work that is never finished and repetitive work
+ Lack of direction
+ Poor time management
+ Holding on – trying to do it all yourself and not using support
+ Inability to make meaningful decisions
+ Inability to feel as though you are 'taking charge' of your life

Are you a candidate for burnout?
+ Are you easily impatient?
+ Are you anxious to maintain your image at all costs?
+ Are you a perfectionist?
+ Do you thrive under pressure?
+ Are people awed by your busy schedule?
+ Are you the pillar of strength and support to others?
+ Are you irritated by silly chitchat?
+ Is being well liked important to you?
+ Do you love responsibility?

As a woman, you are a candidate for burnout! Sure, there are many men who suffer from burnout, but as a woman in South Africa do not underestimate the load you carry. But you can choose to 'burn in' rather than 'burn out'. To 'burn in' means to replenish your internal resources continually, thereby creating energy and vitality.

Take action
Sleep deeply
There are many disturbances to your sleep including your workload, child-rearing, hormonal changes, life events and stressors, but most importantly your mental state. An agitated mind will not allow you to fall asleep easily and will wake you long before you have had adequate, healing sleep.

Sleep has an enormous restorative capacity. During sleep the energy requirements for your muscles, nerves and organs are much lower, so all energy is available for repair processes. This allows your immune system to mop up foreign material and damaged cells and DNA to repair itself. It allows regeneration of cells in your skin and gut and your entire body. This happens all the time but to a much greater degree when you are sleeping. Hormones are also released.

A very important hormone released in greater amounts during sleep is the growth hormone. That is why, as a child, your mom was not lying to you when she said you must go to sleep if you want to grow taller! In children, increased growth hormone released during sleep initiates growth, in fully grown adults it facilitates healing and repair.

Regular exercise, nourishing diet and stress relieving techniques are all factors that enhance sleep (see page 186). Create a sleep transition pattern (at least for most nights of the week) including gearing down, avoiding stimulants and taking a warm bath or shower before easing into bed.

The obvious starting point for managing your stress and improving your energy levels is to develop a consistent, healthy sleep routine. Insomnia or poor-quality sleep is one of the first indications of mental strain. Almost always the cause is internal tension. Even when you do manage to stay asleep, you often wake up groggy and irritable, with the previous day's traumas now deeply embedded into your body and your psyche. Sedative sleeping pills are only justifiable for short periods of time. They are highly addictive with a profound depressant effect.

Most importantly, you need to begin to listen to your body and your fatigue signals. You need to understand your own unique sleep pattern and what works best for you.

Breathe deeply

Deep breathing is such an easy exercise and is a natural tranquilliser for your nervous system. Deep breaths have the capacity to influence your health and healing. Dr Andrew Weil, a medical doctor and author of *Spontaneous Healing*, explains that the single most effective relaxation technique is the conscious regulation of your breath.

Breathing is the only body function that you can control voluntarily. Imagine trying to hold your heartbeat or your gastric acid release for a moment or two? These are impossible to control, but you can control your breath.

By consciously changing the rhythm and depth of your breathing, you can regulate your heart rate, blood pressure, circulation and digestion. This ability to regulate your breath consciously is a powerful mechanism you seldom use. It can profoundly influence your mind, your body and your moods. Deep breathing activates relaxation centres in your brain.

Breathing exercises are very simple, take very little time and can be done almost anywhere. The simplest way is to breathe with the diaphragm and your abdominal muscles. The diaphragm is a muscle that separates your chest cavity from your abdomen and is an important muscle used for breathing. You simply breathe in deeply, filling up your entire lungs, and then slowly, as you breathe out, pull your abdomen (using the abdominal muscles) inwards. You can choose to breathe gently and release strain in those sporadic moments in the day such as standing in the bank and supermarket queues, waiting for a client or school lift or sitting at the robot.

Breathing is also a spiritual practice. Most mystics have identified breath as the cycle that straddles the border between material and non-material reality. In many languages the word for 'breathe' and the word for 'spirit' are identical (Latin *spiritus*, Greek *pneum*, Sanskrit *prana*, Hebrew *neshama*).

You can learn effective breathing techniques in experiences as diverse as yoga, Pilates or meditation or even birth preparation classes. Implementing some simple breathing exercises into your day will go a long way to begin energising your life.

Meditate

You may wonder why it is not good enough just to collapse on the couch at the end of the day in front of the television. Relaxing only your body is not sufficient to combat stress as your mind continues to trigger the outpouring of adrenaline. Research has revealed that the most powerful forms of stress management and relaxation are techniques that still the mind. More and more doctors are prescribing meditation as a way to lower blood pressure, improve exercise performance in people with angina, help people with asthma to breathe more easily, relieve insomnia and generally relax the everyday stresses of life. Meditation is a safe and simple way to balance your physical, emotional and mental states (see page 254).

The basic practice of meditation is amazingly simple. It involves deciding how to direct your mind for a period of time and then doing it. The tedious work of meditation is a constant running after your attention and gently bringing it back to a focus point. For many keen individuals it is so new, so still and so vague an experience that in a very short time it is abandoned. There is no instant gratification, no sweat build-up as after a good workout, no highs as after a delicious chocolate cappuccino. Yet the cumulative effects of meditation are much more profound than any of these could ever be.

During meditation your body is shifted into a parasympathetic-relaxed state during which your blood pressure is reduced, circulation is enhanced, breathing deepens, muscles relax and the immune and endocrine metabolism is improved. Healing, repair and regeneration start to occur.

The mental effects are even more wondrous: agitation and anxiety begin to melt away, depression lifts and genuine self-awareness develops. The practice of meditation allows you to remove a veil and see yourself with some degree of objectivity. With a regular meditation practice, the cumulative effect allows you to tune into a 'quiet' zone that you never knew existed. You begin to develop an exquisite clarity about yourself, your loved ones and the world around you. You begin to feel more energised.

The fact that it may also be a deeply spiritual practice should not put you off if you are not spiritually inclined. The physical and mental benefits are good enough reason to use this technique. If you desire spiritual connectedness, meditation is the obvious starting point, as it allows access to your inner reservoir of infinite potential. Just as you are continually surrounded by a sea of oxygen of which you may be unaware, so too are you oblivious of the sea of spirituality embracing you. Meditation opens up the channels, allowing you to become conscious of this spiritual 'ocean' (see Chapter 6).

With all these remarkable benefits you wonder why most people are not regularly meditating. There are two common reasons. The first is that many are sceptical because they misinterpret meditation as purely Eastern or New Age. On the contrary, it is merely a technique with vast applications ranging from Standardised Clinical Meditation (SCM) used by psychotherapists as a stress management tool, right through the spectrum of religious practice.

The second and more significant reason for its limited practice is that in our fast-paced 21st century, it is very difficult to sit in solitude and quiet for any length of time.

Visualise
Guided imagery
You may find it easier to use a more structured reflective technique, such as guided imagery or visualisation, as it is often called. It can either be performed by a qualified therapist in a one-on-one session or you can use available tapes or CDs. You simply listen to a narrative accompanied by beautiful music that guides you into a state of relaxation. Many people today use creative imagery with tremendous success to improve their lives in a variety of different ways.

Apart from stress management and improved energy levels, guided imagery is being used to combat cancer, pain and chronic illness, improve surgical and maternity outcomes, enhance libido in sexual dysfunction, lift depression and anxiety, assist with peak athletic performance, increase business performance and serve as a tool for learning dysfunction and enhanced school achievement. Guided imagery also causes the release of endorphins in the body.

Medical and scientific research has revealed that imagery can influence your physical body and biochemistry. The body converts images and expectations into biochemical realities through these pathways. Brain centres are stimulated, which in turn send signals to the limbic system (the feeling centre of our brain), the autonomic nervous system (which controls our bodily functions like heart rate, blood pressure) and the endocrine system, the control centre for our hormones, including stress hormones such as cortisol and adrenalin.

Images are not thoughts, they are powerful mental pictures that can be transformed into your reality. Imagery is simply a technique whereby these images are deeply imprinted so that they trigger a cascade of physical and mental effects.

Practical Plan 𝒌

𝒌
Month 5:
Take action
with energy

Week 1:
Rest and sleep
𝒌

OVER THE NEXT few weeks incorporate just one of the following strategies each week:

Rest

Rest is the logical antidote to fatigue, but South African women feel so guilty about resting. Carrying the responsibility of rearing children, contributing to the community and doing a good job of work wears you out. You have to listen to your fatigue signals and build into your day and your week moments to rest!

Begin to listen to your fatigue signals before you burn out. If you cannot find the time during your busy week, you need to make a conscious choice to incorporate resting into your life plan, obviously not every day, but when you feel those lids drooping. If you are in an office all day (even if you are the boss) you could shut your eyes, breathe deeply, meditate or catch a 10-minute catnap during a tea break. You can do this even if you work in an open-plan space. People may think you are strange at first but eventually they will respect you and possibly join you!

If you work from home, you can unquestionably take a rest period during your slump. And don't feel guilty about it! You often make your life busier than it is by not stepping off the roller coaster for a few moments a day to rest.

If there is no way to catch up on rest during the week, give yourself time on the weekend to either sleep in late or have an afternoon rest. If you cannot find any rest periods at all in your week, take two-minute breaks frequently. Leave your desk or office or home and go outdoors – inhale, stretch, smell a flower, touch the grass, exhale and go back to what you were doing. It is remarkable what a difference these few moments of rest will do for your creativity, your energy and especially for those puffy patches under your eyes!

Sleep strategy

Get into a good night time routine. Gear down. Focused work at night stimulates your mind and keeps you 'buzzing' for hours. Have a warm bath and a warm drink before retiring.

Avoid

✦ Focused work or high stimulus television at night.
✦ Stimulants: caffeine contained in coffee, Coke, energy drinks or tonics.

Do

✦ Aerobic exercise at least three times a week (see Chapter 4).
✦ Indulge in a warm bedtime bath with aromatherapy oil. Camomile or lavender oil work best.
✦ Eat a starchy snack 30 minutes prior to bedtime. This releases natural sedatives from your brain, called tryptophan.
✦ Try and create a routine for your sleep pattern at least from Monday to Friday (e.g. get to sleep by 10.30 p.m. and wake by 6.30 a.m.). Your body physiology gets used to the pattern.
✦ Breathing exercises (see below).

◌⋆
Week 2:
Breathe
⋆◌

Breathing

You do this automatically: Fill your lungs with oxygen and blow out carbon dioxide up to twenty times every minute! Now its time to breathe **consciously and slowly**. Deep breathing is such an easy exercise and is one of the most powerful and easiest techniques. Conscious slow breathing literally activates relaxation centres in your brain (see page 225).

1. Observe your breath

Focus on your breathing without trying to influence it in any way. By simply focusing on your breathing, your body

automatically begins to shift into relaxation (parasympathetic response). It is a way to harmonise your body, mind
and spirit.

2. *Start with exhalation*
Breathing is continuous with no beginning and no end, but
you tend to think of inhalation as the beginning. You have
more control during exhalation (out breath) because you
use your voluntary intercostal muscles. You thereby automatically inhale more air, oxygenating your entire body.

3. *Let yourself be breathed*
Imagine with each inspiration the Universe is blowing
breath into you and with each exhalation, withdrawing it.
You are the passive recipient of breath. As the Universe
breathes into you, feel the breath penetrating and healing
every part of your body. This exercise is almost a visualisation technique.

4. *Stimulating breath*
Place the tip of your tongue behind your front teeth.
Breathe in and out rapidly through your nose with your
mouth loosely shut. Start with just 15 seconds and each
time increase by five seconds until you get to a full minute.
This is a real exercise and you can expect to feel fatigue of
some muscles. You can also expect to feel a subtle but defi-
nite movement of energy through the body.

5. *Relaxing breath*
With your tongue in the same position as for 'Stimulating
breath' (above), inhale through your nose to a count of
four, then hold the breath for a count of seven, then exhale
audibly through the mouth for a count of eight. Repeat for
a total of four cycles.
    Begin using these exercises at least once a day and then
increase to a few times each day, particularly when you feel

anxious or unable to sleep. You will probably find that just one of the above works best for you.

(Breathing exercises adapted from 'Spontaneous Healing' by Dr Andrew Weil.)

᯽

Week 3:
Meditation,
Relaxation and
Visualisation

᯽

Meditate

You may choose to learn a formal meditation technique in the near future, but for the time being you can begin by following these instructions (see different meditations in Chapter 6):

1. Find a quiet place to become your meditation spot.
2. Take your phone off the hook, put your mobile onto voicemail, close your door, ask not to be disturbed for the next five or 10 minutes, kids out of bounds.
3. Sit quietly for five minutes. Close your eyes. Sit upright on a chair, or lean on a bed, or sit on the floor.
4. Choose a word or an image as your mantra, for example, a candle flame as an image or the word 'One'.
5. Keep focused on the image or word. If it is a word, mouth the word and repeat over and over, slowly and softly at first.
6. As soon as thoughts enter your mind do not fight them but gently 'sweep them away' with an imaginary broom and bring your attention back to the mantra.
7. That's it! Do not try too hard.
8. Do this for five minutes each day for the next few days.
9. Increase your meditation time to 10 minutes. Do not expect any dramatic changes. The effects are cumulative and subtle at first. But if you build this into your routine the effects on your mind, emotions and spirit will become significant.
10. Try to sit with your mantra for a full 15 minutes. If you are struggling with this, turn on some gentle relaxation music before you start and leave it on very softly while you meditate.

Progressive relaxation

This is based on a simple exercise, comparing tension with relaxation. You sit quietly and then begin the process. It is always good to start with a few deep breaths. You begin by contracting a muscle forcefully for a second or two and then give way to a feeling of relaxation. You start at the top of your head and then go through all the muscle groups one by one, from your neck, your shoulders, your arms, your back, your abdomen, your buttocks, your legs until you lastly get to your feet. The procedure goes through all the muscle groups progressively producing a feeling of total relaxation.

Guided imagery or visualisation

This usually requires either a one on one session or a recording of a guided meditation or visualisation with or without music. This is often much easier than standard meditation as you have the direction of the voice taking you through the relaxation and healing.

𝒦
Week 4:
Pace your life

Understand body
rhythms
𝒦

In practice, how do you begin to flow with your biological rhythms? You would do well to become conscious of your own energy patterns. What times of the day are best or worst for your energy? What sleep times work best for you? Some general guidelines are:

1. Plan important meetings, crucial business negotiations and creative endeavours for first thing in the morning when you are most resilient to stress due to high circulating levels of the antistress hormones.
2. Plan to eat a fairly hearty or sustaining meal at midday, since at midday digestion is most effective.
3. Develop a healthy sleep routine. This is essential to your body rhythms.
4. Track your energy levels. Stop and measure your level of energy at three key times during the day:
   ★ after you wake up in the morning

★ mid-afternoon ± 4 p.m.
★ evening ± 8 p.m.

To determine your level of energy sit quietly and mentally note your energy level on a scale from 1-10. Circle the number on the scale that most represents your energy level:
0 = No energy, complete fatigue
5 = Equal amounts of fatigue and energy
10 = Complete energy and vitality.

At the end of the week connect your circles and see if there is a trend. In another colour, circle any other time in the day that you feel filled with vitality and make a note of what you have just done. Eaten a healthy snack, heard good news, received a compliment, bought something for yourself, completed a meditation?

By using this chart you can become aware of what your body is experiencing and you can begin to eliminate the imbalances that are the basis of chronic fatigue. You will also see the progress as you continue to implement new and healthy techniques into your lifestyle.

CHAPTER 6

Enrich

Introduction

To enrich yourself is to expand, to improve, to advance, to progress and mostly to become deeper. Enrichment is the final phase of your health plan. This chapter will help you challenge and grow your spiritual muscle.

You may ask: *'Why the concept of spirituality here in the midst of a health book?'* Although this book is rooted in medical science, in this final chapter I will digress somewhat from pure science. Your soul defies scientific definition, but I believe it is so central to your physical health that it needs to be incorporated into your health plan. Even though your spirit cannot be dissected in the same way as your anatomy and cannot even be mapped with high-tech brain scans like your emotions or thoughts, it is real and it is powerful.

There has been a dramatic transformation in the world view of medicine and the functioning of the human body. This has taken place against a global shift in thinking. Although there are still those who are reluctant to embrace this new world view, most medical professionals have accepted and supported at least some of the principles of this paradigm. I believe that there have been specific phases of this transformation in health.

The first phase of this new paradigm, which has evolved over the past 30 years, is the role of *prevention* in healthcare and disease management. The responsibility of a patient to make lifestyle adjustments and implement preventive measures is an accepted mainstream medical approach. It was not so 40 years ago! The doctors made all the decisions for their patients and treated their illnesses. There was no conclusive evidence that *you* could prevent disease. And the power and responsibility for health-care resided totally with the doctor.

The second phase is the increasing acceptance of the *integration* of mind and emotions into health and medicine. An example of this is the fact that almost all doctors accept as a basic notion the role that stress plays in the development of heart attacks and stomach ulcers. And then there is a wealth of reliable medical research into the new science of 'mind and body' and the 'emotions and physiology'. These areas have come to the fore and have almost become mainstream thinking for many people.

I propose that the third phase of this paradigm is the concept that the physical body and its spiritual counterparts are *interrelated*. This sounds like a fairly alternative perspective and obviously not everyone will accept this view. The very nature of spirituality will always pose more questions than answers and defies science and definition. There is no doubt, how-ever, that we have experienced a worldwide awakening to spirituality. People are feeling the need for a spiritual connection.

Spirituality, however, is not a central tenet in a Western medical model. And perhaps never can be. The reason for this is that the practice of medicine is evidence-based. Understandably, you dare not use a medi-cation or surgical technique that has not been scientifically proven.

But do science and the mystical intersect at any point? Is medicine purely a science or is the art of healing an important aspect? At the core of healing is a deep spiritual component comprising faith, belief, hope, prayer and the unknown. If these aspects are completely incompatible with Western science, then we are saying that medicine and healing are mutually exclusive. I think not! I think that healing is fundamental to healthcare. Medical people may be afraid to use terms such as spiritual-ity, belief systems, miracles and prayer, and instead talk of social support and spontaneous remission. This is just a matter of terminology. The fun-damentals of this connection of spirituality with health and healing are not new at all but are rooted in thousands-year-old ancient healing path-ways whose principles are vital and relevant to the 21st century. Although much of the information within this book is based on scientific data, the particulars within this chapter are primarily drawn from these spiritual wisdoms.

Spirituality can be felt and expressed in so many different ways. And they are all valuable and meaningful. For some women spirituality is expressed through the structure of religion and formal prayer services. For others it may be through a sense of belonging within a community and reaching out with meaningful actions. So many people today prefer a less formal or rigid framework. For many, the world of spirit and meaning is found in nature, in wildlife, in hiking through the mountains or near the ocean. The world of spirituality and godliness is everywhere within you, around you, beyond you, and your expression of spirituality can be any one of these or all at the same time. On your journey through life, you will move through different experiences and expressions of this dimension within you.

You are a spiritual being, no matter how physical you may seem. These dimensions are interconnected within you. In healthcare, the concept of spirituality seems to emerge only with the care of dying patients, when even medical personnel encourage their patients to connect with and express a sense of spirituality. You do not need to wait until the end of your life to acknowledge, to feed and to grow your soul dimension. My belief as a mainstream Western medical doctor is that although it cannot be measured, your spirituality and its impact on your health is enormous.

Precious's story (and my story)

The older I get the more 'precious' this incident becomes. It has remained with me for nearly 20 years. What I realise now many years later is that often dying people not only teach us the most about spirituality, but they also have enormous power to heal us. Precious, an elderly, dignified woman, was one of the very first patients I ever examined as a medical student fresh into my first clinical block. I met Precious at the enormous Baragwanath (Chris Hani Memorial) Hospital in the mid-1980s. My group of students were assigned to Precious as she had overt clinical signs that were easy to examine and apparently useful for our education – a massively enlarged liver and huge palpable lymph nodes throughout her body. She was extremely ill and I remember her unexpectedly serene face in stark contrast to the oppressive November heat, the stench of bedpans, and most of all my intense fear of a dying patient.

After all eight of us had finished our turn at prodding and poking, our teacher, the surgeon, returned to conduct the tutorial. He somehow thought this an opportune time (perhaps he misguidedly thought breaking harsh news was part of our edification) to share the news. He proceeded to tell Precious that unfortunately there was nothing more that could be done for her medically, and perhaps she'd better start praying. I suddenly felt that familiar dizzy feeling that would accompany me right through medical school, whenever I was about to faint.

As all the students uncomfortably pulled away from the bedside – a trail of white coats following our teacher to the next case – I collapsed onto the stool next to Precious, placing my head between my legs, and immediately felt a tug on my arm and a whisper to my ear. I had assumed incorrectly that she could not speak English very well. She told me in a soft whisper that yes, she was praying but not for a cure as the doctor meant. She told me not to be upset because she has already seen her 'ancestors' and her beloved family on the other side in her dreams night after night in the hospital. She was at peace and was praying to them to accompany her on her journey to the next life.

The full meaning and impact of this lesson was not apparent to me as a 19-year-old student. But it has unfolded profoundly in 20 years. I learned that teachers come in unexpected guises and that spiritual lessons for a lifetime can be received in just a few minutes. Although deeply appreciative of my training and my teachers, seven years of medical school and countless academics could not have taught me the following:

+ I learnt from Precious in that moment that prayer does not mean getting what we want and in our way.
+ I learnt that prayer may be more about letting go and trusting than begging for a miracle.
+ I learnt my first lesson in not fearing death.
+ I learnt in those few brief moments about the comfort of staying close to your spiritual tradition and belief system.

✦ I also learnt most profoundly that healing does not necessarily mean curing. Precious was riddled with cancer but died perfectly healed.
✦ Most of all, I was fortunate to receive healing and comfort (surprisingly from a dying patient) as well as some of her profound African spiritual wisdom.

Spirituality and medicine

When you walk into your doctor's office, you bring much more than a headache or chest pain. Patients carry with them not only their thoughts and emotions but also ideas about their belief systems. For years physicians did not consider how such factors as spirituality affected patients' health or their responses to medical treatment. The reality is that they were just not taught. Today countless prestigious medical schools are including *spiritual medicine* in their mainstream teaching curriculum.

At the turn of the 20th century, scientific medicine and spiritual medicine butted heads. It was one or the other. Scientific medicine reigned supreme. The mechanistic model and technology in medicine has translated into incredible advancement in the treatment of disease. However, today medicine needs to use both spiritual and allopathic treatment. Medical professionals *do* need to address the spiritual needs of a patient. This does not mean that your doctor can actually *meet* your spiritual needs but he or she does need to *address* them as part of your health management. You need to meet your own spiritual needs for the good of your health.

Throughout history, religion and spirituality and the practice of medicine have been intertwined. As a result, many religions embrace caring for the sick as a primary mission and many of the world's leading medical institutions have religious and spiritual roots. A recent survey of a huge number of family physicians found that 96 per cent believe that spiritual wellbeing is an important factor in health. Despite these findings, the spiritual needs of patients are often ignored. Medical interest in spiritual health has increased mainly because of a growing number of convincing studies that have shown an association between spiritual involvement and better health outcomes.

A Mayo Clinic academic review of 1200 valid clinical studies which have used religious and spiritual variables in assessing health was conducted recently. This body of research demonstrates that religious involvement and spirituality are associated with better health outcomes. The mechanisms by which religious involvement and spirituality affect health are not always understood. These mechanisms undoubtedly involve complex interactions of psychosocial and behavioural factors on biological processes, as well as immeasurables such as belief and the supernatural.

The studies have shown that religious involvement and spirituality are associated with greater longevity, better coping skills and much improved health-related quality of life (even during terminal illness). The studies also demonstrate less anxiety, depression and suicide. Most importantly, several studies have shown that addressing the spiritual needs of the patient may enhance recovery from illness.

Spirituality and your health

Like many of the other health promoting practices discussed in this book, such as exercise, spirituality is likely to enhance your resistance to disease by the interaction of multiple beneficial factors. Religiously involved or spiritually inclined people are more likely to choose healthier lifestyles. They follow a nutritious diet, seek preventive healthcare and avoid risky behaviour such as smoking. They are also more involved in strong social support systems (the healing benefits of which have been discussed earlier in this book). But these factors do NOT account for all the health benefits of spirituality. Recent prospective studies have adjusted for these factors in their research and have still found a significant relationship between spirituality and positive health outcomes. Hence other factors must be responsible for the benefits.

Spiritual practices, such as meditation and prayer, engender positive emotions, such as hope, love, contentment and forgiveness, and limit negative emotions, such as hostility and despair. The positive emotions can lead to decreased activity of the sympathetic branch of your autonomic nervous system and the hormone control to your adrenal gland. This leads to reduced release of stress hormones such as adrenalin and cortisol. This response has psychological effects (less anxiety) and physiological effects (decreased heart rate and blood pressure) and these may lead to better health. Spiritually involved people also demonstrate an enhanced immune function. And so much that we cannot measure.

Spiritually-based medicine can be better termed a medicine of meaning. Spiritual medicine is not as separate from science as you would imagine. It is consistent with quantum physics and is rooted in the belief that we live in a vast, interconnected, interdependent world.

What is soul?

Your soul defies definition and measurement but there are many ways to describe it. It is your unique personality, your essential being. Although it is intangible and deeply embedded within you, it is your soul that energises your body. It is the core of your humanity.

Philosophers argue about what to call this core of your humanity. Buddhists call it original nature, Quakers call it the inner teacher, Humanists call it identity. In Greek it is *pneum*, in Sanskrit it is *prana*, in Hebrew it is *nefesh*. In the Sotho language in South Africa we call it *moya*. What you name it matters little, but that you name it matters a great deal.

Where soul meets body

The functions of your physical body and its spiritual counterpart may be totally interrelated. Though physical, your human body reflects levels of spirituality. Your soul is manifest in every part of your anatomy.

How do you unite soul and body? How do you integrate the sacred and the mundane, the spiritual and the material? Jewish mysticism addresses this issue with what is called the 'cosmic order' which consists of a series of stepping stones uniting spirit and matter.

There are many layers to reality. The physical world as you know it is just the surface level, within which exist many dimensions of spiritual energy. Every material element, particularly your physical body, is invested with a higher, more spiritual one. (Water, for example, is the physical embodiment of love and kindness, while fire represents the physical dimension of power.)

You are certainly able to see the physical outer layers of reality, but may struggle to glimpse into the spiritual essence that lies within you. And yet God has enabled you to peel back the successive layers of the container – that is your body – to reveal the inner glow. And when you do peel these layers by nourishing, exercising and energising your soul, you then raise your sensitivity to the spiritual forces within and the by-product of this is spiritual wellbeing and healing.

Soul in your anatomy

There is a very interesting concept explained in Jewish Mysticism (*Kabbala*) that describes the qualities of spirituality as embedded within the physical body. Ten qualities of spirituality or godliness are described, as represented in the human body. This idea portrays each quality as residing within a part of the anatomy. The human physical body containing these spiritual qualities is called the *Tree of Life*. This may be referred to in other wisdoms as the 'cosmic body'. Every aspect of life is comprised of a right, left and centre. For example, your right brain, left brain and middle brain.

Your entire body is structured in three columns: the right side (right arm and leg), the left side (left arm and leg) and the centre (the spine), which creates balance. The Tree of Life is also divided into these three columns: right, left and centre. These ten powers or spiritual qualities include glory, wisdom, understanding, loving kindness, strength, harmony, empathy, endurance, foundation of energy and humility. The right brain, right arm and right leg comprise the right column. The left brain, left arm and left leg comprise the left column. The centre column is made up of the crown, the spine and torso and the base of the body, including the genitalia. Harmony is the centre column that runs a direct line from one end, which is the crown of the head, to the other end in the base of the spine and genitalia. From the top down, these qualities are described in the human body as follows:

1. Glory = Crown of the head, cranium
2. Wisdom = Right brain
3. Understanding = Left brain
4. Loving kindness = Right arm

5. Strength and discipline =
   Left arm
6. Harmony, balance = Torso
7. Empathy = Right leg
8. Endurance and
   containment = Left leg
9. Foundation of energy =
   Base of spine, genitalia
10. Humility = Female
    genitalia

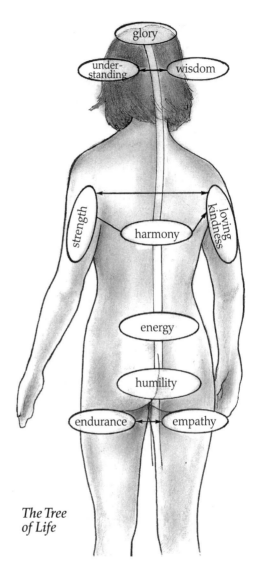

I have shared this concept with you not only as an interesting and stimulating spiritual idea but also because I think it can have some practical application in living a healthy and balanced life. Often the missing ingredient in your life that may be responsible for your illnesses, your low moods or your fatigue is a lack of harmony.

The quality of harmony represents the power to integrate all the opposing energies. In the Tree of Life you need to balance loving kindness with strength and discipline, empathy with containment and glory with humility. The opposing aspects in your life that don't seem to fit together include faith and doubt, the spiritual and the physical, male and female, strength and vulnerability, love and discipline, and especially your body and soul. Just like the right and left sides of your body and brain require a central stabilising quality called

The Tree of Life

your spine, your Tree of Life needs this harmony or balance to contain your spiritual qualities. This power of balance will help you suspend your ego, your perspective, your perceptions, your fears and doubts, and allow yourself to be a channel for something far greater than yourself.

Your soul as energy

In continuing to describe the soul, it is vital that you consider the concept of energy. The entire universe is a field of energy that surrounds us. Einstein revealed through quantum physics that every atom in the universe is in constant motion and is interconnected into a unified, energetic field.

Although your soul is unable to be measured by the instrumentation of modern physics, it too is composed of waves of energy which are connected to a universal field of vibrating energy waves and particles. The closest that scientists can get to some type of measurement is in quantifying the magnetic energetic field immediately surrounding your body. This field of energy outside of your body may be one of the layers of what is commonly called (in spiritual circles) your aura, described as a colour or light that surrounds you. You certainly have a magnetic field surrounding your body which can be measured. The aura and you magnetic field may be one and the same.

If you suffer from fatigue as a symptom of a medical condition, depression or chronic fatigue syndrome, it is worth considering the deficiency or imbalance of spiritual energy as just one of many factors that need to be addressed.

Your soul: within or without, above or below?

We seem to think of our soul as embedded within us and in order to connect with it, we need to dig deep within. There is no doubt that your spiritual nature is somewhere within, but it is somewhere outside of you, too. The aspects of this external soul dimension may be found in the magnetic field or aura that surrounds your physical body, or the spiritual energy or light around your head described as your crown chakra in Hinduism, or the crown dimension in the Tree of Life.

Your soul exists not only within, but also without – it is your spiritual signature. The people and places touched by your soul are imprinted with your essence. Everywhere you go, you leave behind the valuable, unique signature of your soul.

Just as your body is a whole unified system made up of interconnected elements, so too your soul contains different parts. There is a soul within and a soul without, but there is also a description of a soul above and a soul below. The soul below is sometimes called the 'animal soul'. This is the animating force of your physical body, governing and closely connected to your growth, development and physical functioning, as well as your instincts, feelings, intelligence and imagination. Linked to this, but far more exalted, is the soul above or the 'divine soul' which connects you to the highest planes. The divine soul is the channel through which 'spirituality' is transmitted to you. From the divine soul these influences are then transmitted via the animal soul to your physical body. Thus the divine soul is clothed in the animal soul and the animal soul is clothed in the body.

The divine soul in fact consists of different levels bound together like links in a chain. In the same way as the links form one chain, these levels of soul form a single entity. The five components from the top down are referred to as *unique essence, living essence, breath essence, spirit, and animal soul*. Each of these levels is bound to the one below until the lowest one (animal soul) is bound to the body.

From all these descriptions, you can begin to understand that your soul is intricately connected with your body, and spiritual pursuits will indeed add to your total health.

What is spirituality?

Spirituality is an awareness of the divine or sacred core that underlies everyday life. It is a belief system focusing on intangible elements that bring vitality and meaning to your life's events. Religion and spirituality are among the most important factors that give structure and meaning to your human values and experiences. In global surveys, most people report having a spiritual life. Surveys done on both patient groups and the general population have consistently found that more than 90 per cent of people believe in a Higher Being. One such survey found that 94 per cent of patients regard their spiritual health and their physical health as equally important. The most impressive result for me is that 96 per cent of family physicians believe that spiritual wellbeing is an important factor in health.

Even though many people who regard themselves as spiritual do not endorse a formal religion, religious involvement and spirituality are certainly overlapping concepts.

Universal spiritual principles: the things that bind us

There are accepted wisdoms that traverse every belief system, golden strands that run through the fibre of every religion, faith and creed. These golden strands are identical in each system. But because they are named different things, far more attention is placed on the discrepancies and divergences than the commonality and connectedness of all people. Regardless of religious separations and disparities, these are potent aspects of life that are common to all. The four principles of spirituality that are shared by all belief systems include:

1. **Purpose:** There is a real purpose in your life. Each human is unique and has a specific purpose on earth.
2. **Connectedness:** Human beings are connected. You have many levels of connection: connection to loved ones, connections in intimacy, connections in the workplace, connections to your community, your culture and to the world around you. You need these connections with others in order to thrive.
3. **Transcendence:** You have the capacity to go beyond yourself. What this means is that you are capable of reaching out to others and making a real difference in acts of compassion, loving kindness, charity and social responsibility. Transcendence also means you have the capacity to go beyond your self-imposed limitations, your suffering and your pain.
4. **Belief:** The majority of people have a belief in a Force greater than themselves.

Spirituality for non-believers

There is a well-known story about a famous 18th-century spiritual master, the Baal Shem Tov (translated his name means 'the owner of a good name'), who was renowned for his empathy and non-judgmental character. One holy festival he invited his neighbour to come with him to his place of worship. The neighbour declined, saying, _'Master, I'm an atheist, I don't believe in God. It would be hypocritical of me to set foot in your place of worship.'_ The great master smiled and replied, _'The God that you don't believe in, I don't believe in either.'_

Notwithstanding this parable, there are certainly agnostics, atheists and many people who seriously doubt the existence of a spiritual dimension. But even without a formal belief in God, there is a 'humanness' that may at some point intersect with the concept of spirituality.

The description of greatness in a human being would encompass many positive character traits and achievements. I would ascribe just four concepts to many of the world's greatest human beings from Mother Theresa to Nelson Mandela:

1. The presence of a _profound life purpose_
2. A _sense of connectedness_ to people
3. The _ability to transcend_ limitations and suffering
4. A _belief_ in something greater than oneself.

The four principles of spirituality are indeed the selfsame principles of human greatness.

Healing

I now put my medical hat back on to share with you something absolutely fascinating. Much research has been done on cancer sufferers and seriously ill patients, trying to determine why some people unexpectedly recover. What are some of the factors that contribute to their surprising results?

In so many instances a patient defies the doctor's bleak prognosis and medical science's predictions. These cases used to be called miracles. They are far too common now to be labeled miracles, so medical science has given them a name, _'spontaneous remissions'_. Healing is perhaps the point where medicine meets spirituality. It is also the point where your body meets your soul.

There are certain common features to be found in patients who experience spontaneous remissions or unexpected healing. Among a host of common factors, the following four features are present in many of these patients:

1. **Purpose:** People who undergo spontaneous remissions almost always feel a profound sense of purpose in their lives. Much research in the field of psycho-oncology (cancer and psychology) reveals that survival itself depends on seeking and finding meaning and purpose. It is clear that many people cope more easily with the challenges of illness if they recognise that life has a deep sense of meaning. Purpose, together with passion, seems to fire up the immune system producing active immune substances to ward off illness, mop up damaged cells and augment the body's healing. Amazingly, physical healing sometimes takes place as a direct result of the passion and purpose with which you live. It builds a reservoir of physical and emotional power enabling you to withstand your stresses and sorrows.

2. **Connection:** People with a strong support system, where love can be expressed and received, have a much higher incidence of spontaneous remissions and healing than those without this. Much scientific evidence exists and continues to grow in medical literature on the health damaging consequences of loneliness and isolation, and the life-enhancing power of love, support and connections.

3. **Going beyond:** Those patients who can reach beyond themselves and transcend their suffering are most likely to experience unexpected healing. These are patients who look for ways to reach out. It does not mean that they do not feel the pain or suffering. Transcendence simply means they do not get stuck, but move beyond their pain.

4. **Belief:** Almost 100 per cent of patients who undergo spontaneous remissions and unexpected recovery in other studies, hold a belief in a Supreme Being.

My humble observation in the realm of spontaneous remissions or miracle cures is that these people are demonstrating spiritual qualities and are living soulful lives. There is so much beyond understanding. This does not mean that you have a formula to healing yourself. It is a simple observation. The four principles that comprise spirituality are the same principles that are present in human greatness and are once again the same features found in unexpected healing. These are truly universal principles to aspire to as the rules for meaningful and healthy living.

However, it is important to understand that if you are seriously ill and living with an incurable illness it does **not** mean that you are **not** living a spiritual, soulful life. We cannot understand the full picture of the Universe, particularly in the realm of illness. Many factors are way beyond human grasp. The concept of healing is so much more than curing or fixing (see discussion in Chapter 1). Healing comes from two words which embody its meaning: *whole* and *holy*. To heal is to become a 'whole' integrated human being who has a 'holy' dimension. Obviously, if you are ill, what you want more than anything else is complete physical recovery. But healing does not always mean that the physical body has the capacity to recover 100 per cent from an illness. Healing can also mean that your family and intimate bonds draw closer. It may mean you feel closer to God through your prayers and devotion. It may mean that you are able to transform your fear to courage, your despair to hope, your bitterness to forgiveness and your judgment to compassion.

Very often, when confronted with a serious illness, a person embarks on a healing journey, trying all methods to obtain a cure and achieve wellbeing, and through this a spiritual journey is often evoked. The journey to healing is parallel to an internal soul journey, but you need not wait for a serious illness before connecting with your inner self and embarking on a healing journey.

Spiritual prescription

In medicine, a prescription can be a cure or a form of treatment recommended to correct a problem. Your doctor's prescription also includes advice and information. If you came to me for advice or treatment for your ailment, you would often leave my office with a prescription, commonly called a *script*. You will take leave of this book with a spiritual script, too! This consists of recommended activities and remedies for your spiritual life.

You may require a spiritual script or are drawn to spirituality because you are experiencing many of the common symptoms of a condition which I have termed the 'Spiritual Deficiency Syndrome'. You may feel that something is missing in your life. You could be in pain and in need of healing. You could be thirsting for inspiration. You may be craving a sense of community or even quality time. You could be feeling fairly content and grateful and compelled to give something back. You could be facing a crisis and need to harness your resources. You could simply be burned out and seriously fatigued or you could be worried about your loved ones and their safety. The most common symptom of 'Spiritual Deficiency Syndrome' is a rumbling sense that your life could be more meaningful.

What you require in your script is spiritual practices. These activities are designed to move you into deeper relationships with God, your true self, other people and the environment around you. The difference with this prescription is that I will not prescribe and choose a course of treatment for you. You need to choose these activities yourself. What you choose should be based on what your symptoms may be and what practices you think you need or you will actually do.

Firstly you need to examine your symptoms – what is really happening in your life? For example, if part of your life pain is about being stuck in the past or a past relationship, your spiritual work is to let go and begin to live in the present. If you are fearful, you need to work on trust, if you are lonely you need to practise reaching out to others.

The tools

Just as your body requires nourishment by the best quality foods, dynamic exercise to achieve fitness and strength and energising activity to create vitality, so too your soul requires these three aspects to attain spiritual health.

Your soul prescription contains a three-pronged approach incorporating the nourishment for your soul, the recommended exercise script for your soul and the energising of your soul. The activities of prayer, meditation, acquiring wisdom and virtuous deeds are nourishment, exercise and energy for your soul and thereby your body, too. They are indeed the pillars of spiritual living and are the basis of your spiritual prescription. The health of your body is interdependent with the health of your soul. And it is your responsibility to nurture them both.

Prayer

Although the world may seem huge, diverse and bewildering, prayer is the bridge, the single activity that has the capacity to unite all people, cultures, religious paths and practices. Although so many religious prayers are structured, there isn't just one right way to pray – what works well for one person may not for another. It may be individual or communal, formal or informal. You may find that informal and unstructured prayer is best for you or you may prefer to join other people, who may be gathering to pray in local communities or prayer groups. You may find that you can say just what you want to, using your own words, but many people find it helpful to use written prayers.

The word prayer is derived from the Latin word *precari* which means to ask, to beseech, to implore, to request. The two most common forms of prayer are *petition* – to ask something for yourself – and *intercession* – asking something for others. Other types of prayer are *confession* – the repentance of wrongdoing and asking for forgiveness, *thanksgiving* – offering gratitude, and *adoration* – offering praise.

Prayer, described as a non-local event, has the capacity to reach outside the here and now. It is a time for you to literally nourish your soul. The habit of prayer should not be burdensome, for you can pray worthily at any time, in any place and in any posture. Prayer produces a feeling of hope, and the simple process allows you to flex and stretch your spiritual muscles. The positive health benefit through attendance at religious services was reviewed in a number of medical studies. Those who attended services weekly or more had significantly better health across a vast array of illnesses. Medical researchers went one step further to try and determine which type of prayer works best – *directed prayer* in which prayers have a specific goal or outcome in mind, or *undirected prayer*, in which no specific outcome is requested. Researchers found that while both types of prayer produced results, the undirected approach was quantitatively more effective, frequently yielding results twice as great or more compared to the directed approach. The undirected approach encompassing a 'letting go' and a trust in God facilitates a release, peace and hope.

When it comes to prayer and spirituality, I find one approach problematic and in serious conflict with all my principles as a doctor and a healer. Any religious or spiritual belief system that refuses medical intervention and prefers instead to rely solely on prayer with the outright refusal of therapy especially with regard to children, is negligent and is contravening a spiritual responsibility to take utmost care to safeguard the physical body.

Most of the different belief systems agree that there is an order to effective praying. And the first step in prayer is to *praise* God. Everyone has huge life challenges and I think it is only human when praying to start by asking for God's help in solving problems By giving praise and gratitude first, you shift your focus outside of yourself away from your problem towards God. To praise first is the first step in transcendence. You can learn from this and apply this principle to relationships. It is a real stretching exercise to thank and praise your loved one or your friend first, before diving into a discourse on your problems. (Be creative and make up your own 'mini-prayers'. Keep all your prayers short, simple and centred.)

Meditation
The practice of meditation is not new. The value of meditation to promote healing has been known and practised for thousands of years. The only new thing is the documented medical benefits and the widespread, mainstream use of this very effective technique. Meditative techniques are the product of diverse cultures and have been rooted in the traditions of the world's great religions. Practically all religious groups practise meditation in one form or another.

The basic practice of meditation is amazingly simple. It involves deciding how to direct your mind for a period of time and then doing it. The intention is to direct your concentration to one healing element – one sound, one word, one image or one's breath. All forms of meditation require regular, daily practice over a long period of time before they deliver rewards. It also takes commitment to pursue such a quiet activity.

In addition to the physical and mental benefits (see Chapter 5), you can truly nourish your soul through meditation and at the same time develop genuine self-awareness. The practice allows you to remove a veil and see yourself with some degree of objectivity. It helps you to tune into a 'quiet' zone that you never knew existed. You begin to feel more energised. Just as you are continually surrounded by a sea of oxygen of which you may be unaware, so too are you oblivious of the sea of spirituality embracing you. Meditation opens up the channels, allowing you to become conscious of this spiritual 'ocean'. In essence it is a spiritual practice that can offer you a sense of hope and peace and joy and true closeness to your spirit within and the Spirit without. The longer you practise meditation, the greater the likelihood that your goals and efforts will shift toward personal and spiritual growth. Many individuals who initially learn meditation for its health aspects find that as their practice deepens, they are drawn more and more into the realm of the spiritual.

Types

Of the various different types of meditation, the most commonly practised in Western society are transcendental meditation (TM) and mindfulness meditation. The difference between two basic techniques is:

Concentrative/Transcendental meditation focuses the attention on the breath, an image or a sound – in other words a mantra, in order to still the mind and allow a greater awareness and clarity to emerge. This is like a zoom lens in a camera: you narrow your focus to a selected field. The most commonly practised form of concentrative meditation is transcendental meditation which focuses on a mantra.

Mindfulness meditation, on the other hand can be likened to a wide-angle lens. Instead of narrowing your vision to a selected field as in concentrative meditation, here you are aware of the entire field. It involves becoming aware of the continuously passing parade of feelings, images and thoughts without becoming involved in thinking about them. You sit quietly and simply witnesses whatever goes through your mind, not reacting or becoming involved with them.

How to
1. Find a comfortable spot to use as your regular meditation site. Try to use the same place every day. You will come to associate that place with the serene mood. It does not matter if you sit in a chair, on your bed, a couch or the floor.
2. If you use a word or a mantra it helps at the beginning to mouth the word or whisper it over and over.
3. Do not worry too much about all the thoughts that appear in your head. Gently return to your word or mantra. Sit for five minutes for the first few days and then increase slowly up till 20 minutes each day. If you cannot find a 20-minute slot, use a few five-minute mediations through the day.
4. Do not try too hard!
5. The effects are cumulative, so the most important principle is to keep up the practice consistently. When you skip a day or two, you start losing the effect.
6. Use the few moments following a meditation to have a personal conversation with God. This moment immediately following your meditation is often filled with a feeling of peace and closeness. In some belief systems, meditation is not only regarded as an end in itself, it is also often a preparation for something more, such as prayer.

Spiritual benefits
Feeling safe: You are able to gain a sense that you are not alone in the Universe, even at those times when you feel temporarily separated from other people. You feel increasingly safe as you come to believe that there is a source you can always turn to in times of difficulty.

248

Peace of mind: This is the result of feeling a deep, abiding sense of safety. It is not that you give up your will or are unrealistic; you simply learn that you can 'let go'. To let go when solutions to problems aren't immediately apparent can go a long way towards reducing anxiety in your life.

Self-confidence: You come to realise something good and lovable and worthy of respect within you.

Unconditional love: As you develop a deeper connection with God, you come to experience greater degrees of unconditional love in your life. You feel your heart opening more easily to people. You feel free of judgment towards them. Unconditional love shows up both in your increased capacity to give love to others and to experience more of it coming into your life. You begin to experience less fear and more joy in your life.

Guidance: Developing a connection with your inner self or with God will provide you with guidance for making decisions and solving problems.

Wisdom

Although I have included 'wisdom' in your spiritual prescription, it is not something that can be prescribed. You cannot seek to become 'wise'. But you can seek, accumulate and internalise knowledge. There is huge value in making the time to study from spiritual or religious texts and teachers. But acquiring wisdom is a process that is an integration of knowledge, introspection, the refining of personal qualities, insight and, of course, time. But keep it as a central focus and a goal in your spiritual enrichment.

Knowledge is very powerful. It enables you to take charge of your life and make informed decisions. At a mind-body level, knowledge itself has the capacity to heal. By knowing how something affects your body, the neurochemicals can become structured in your system and can help nourish and energise you. From a spiritual position, acquiring spiritual knowledge literally feeds your soul and energises you. When you are grappling with difficult or new concepts, you exercise, build up and stretch the muscles of your soul.

Although there is so much to be gleaned from many diverse spiritual pathways, it is always worth exploring your own roots first. There is merit in beginning to study the spiritual or religious tradition you were born into as this often resonates with your soul. However, if it doesn't feel right, you have a choice of knowledge you wish to explore. There is value in having guidance or teachers in acquiring this knowledge. Whether they are ministers, priests, rabbis, imams, sages, masters, elders, gurus or regular people, a teacher may play an important part in your spiritual unfolding. In reality, in the spiritual world everything you encounter and everyone you meet is a teacher.

On this path to spiritual wisdom you need to balance your own sense of empowerment closely i.e. your own judgment, with the possible surrendering of your soul to a leader and needing the constant affirmation of your teacher. Seek your teacher's wisdom and knowledge and at the same time develop the confidence to maintain personal responsibility for your spiritual growth and wisdom.

Deeds and actions

We all know the old saying *'Actions speak louder than words'*. In the spiritual dimension, words have enormous power. Words make up the Bible and the written scriptures of all traditions. Words make up the prayers and structure of formal devotion. Words make up psalms and hymns. Most significantly, words are the way in which the physical world was created.

Actions, however, are even more powerful than words. Your actions and deeds provide the light for those around you, but also provide the fuel to feed your own soul. Although it seems that by extending a helping hand through acts of love, compassion and caring you may drain your energy, it spiritually nurtures you, too. Obviously this outward flow always needs to be in a balance with an inward flow of compassion, caring and love to yourself (see Chapter 2).

An important question to ask at this juncture is: What is the point of a spiritual life? You may answer: To connect with Godliness and to develop your soul. I may have even convinced you that the main reason is for the effects on your physical health! But the real value and meaning of a spiritual life is to create 'soul' in the world around you. It is what you do with it – your actions. Once your soul has been nourished and expanded and energised and polished so that it glows, there is no point of the glow alone on a mountain. Use that radiance to light up those around you. Your actions are the internal fuel and the external flame at the same time.

The supplements

Prayer, meditation, acquiring wisdom and virtuous deeds are the main-stay of your spiritual prescription and play a preventive and maintenance role in the health of your soul. But there are additional supplementary requirements for complete spiritual wellbeing. I call these the soul vita-mins, minerals and nutrients.

I have created a symptom chart for you to identify your symptoms and determine which 'nutrient' and practices you most need to fill your spir-itual prescription. Undoubtedly all of these aspects together are necessary for your spiritual wellbeing. This chart is simply a guide to integrate all these aspects into a harmonious balance. There is no way that you can just focus on one specific remedy for one area that needs attention in your spiritual life, but you can pay more attention to an area of weakness in order to restore balance and harmony to your whole spiritual self.

Note: These vitamins and minerals are simply metaphors.

Table 1: Symptom and spiritual supplement chart

Symptom	Spiritual nutrient – spiritual practice
Stress	Vitamin A – Attention, awareness Attention is also known as mindfulness or awareness. Use this spiritual vitamin to stay alert and conscious in your daily life. The good news is that attention can be practised anywhere, any time and in your daily activities. Begin by doing one thing at a time. Focus on your breath whenever you remember to become attentive.
Living in the past	Vitamin B – Being present The spiritual practice of being present means simply that – *present* in the here and now. The *being* is as important as the *present*, i.e. being fully awake and alert and appreciative for this particular place and this particular moment in your life.

continued overleaf

Table 1: Symptom and spiritual supplement chart (continued)

Symptom	Spiritual nutrient – spiritual practice
Separation, loneliness	**Vitamin C – Connections** A delightful definition of spirituality is 'the art of making connections'. Everything is interrelated in time, space and within you. You cannot thrive as a human being and as a woman without your connections to your family, loved ones, community and spirituality. The practice of connections reinforces your awareness of how the spiritual, physical, emotional and mental aspects of your self nourish one another.
Lack of commitment	**Vitamin D – Devotion** It can be any practice you do on a daily basis, including your morning prayers or meditation. Devotion demands a commitment and consistent practice. It is therefore a powerful vitamin that regularly nourishes and connects you to your internal self and to the Divine.
Boredom, lack of meaning	**Vitamin E – Enthusiasm** Enthusiasm is a powerful remedy as it counterbalances apathy and boredom. It is a spiritual vitamin that ignites your passions, allowing you to share your excitement with others. The word is derived from the roots *en* within and *theos* meaning God. It means having God within, and is a quality that encourages you to give outwards and hold back very little. The antidote to exhaustion may not be rest. It may be enthusiasm.
Self-absorbed	**Vitamin K – Loving kindness** This spiritual Vitamin K is the core of religious and spiritual conduct. Loving kindness is a primary quality of an awakened spirit and of a generous human being. This practice means being generous with yourself, your skills, time, money and your resources. True acts of loving kindness are about giving freely without expecting anything in return. Few women would describe themselves as unkind or nasty, yet you and I would have to admit that we often miss the mark on this spiritual practice.
Judgmental	**Ca (calcium) – Compassion** Just as calcium is required throughout your life for the development of strong bones, this spiritual mineral is essential for the strength of your spiritual framework. Allow yourself to feel. Do not turn away from pain; move toward it with caring. It is very good exercise for your heart and your soul muscle.

Table 1: Symptom and spiritual supplement chart *(continued)*

Symptom	Spiritual nutrient – spiritual practice
Bitterness, resentment	**Fe (iron) – Forgiveness** Fe, the scientific symbol for iron, is a trace element which is needed by the body for the formation of blood. Fe deficiency anaemia is probably the commonest nutritional deficiency and the commonest symptom is extreme fatigue. So, too, a lack of the spiritual Fe (forgiveness) mineral leads to a draining of your life force, causing spiritual fatigue. Persistent unforgiveness is part of human nature, but not being able to forgive is detrimental to your spiritual wellbeing and your physical health. Forgiveness does not mean condoning another's hurtful behaviour – it means *letting go* of your own suffering.
Cynical or emptiness	**Mg (magnesium) – Meaning** Meaning is also a specific spiritual practice that can be learned, developed and applied. It involves both the seeking and making life meaningful. Seek meaning by looking at the big picture of your life, but also in the small details. Everything in your life has meaning. To everything there is a purpose, even if it appears to the contrary. If what you are doing doesn't seem important, it's time to work with the practice of meaning. Spend time and energy on the things that are really meaningful to you.
Unfulfilled	**Potassium – Passion** If you are to lead a deep, fulfilling and connected life, then you will require plenty of this mineral. Living passionately gives meaning to every aspect of your life. This synergy between passion and meaning may fire up your immune system, producing active immune substances to augment your body's healing and possibly ward off illness.
Chaos and stress	**Se (Selenium) – Silence** You are bombarded daily with the noise of life. Silence is a powerful antidote. Like selenium, this spiritual nutrient of silence is only needed in small amounts for its powerful effect in preventing and neutralising damage. Set aside a little time alone to be involved in simple introspection. This puts you in control of your life rather than the pace of life controlling you.
Entitlement	**Gamma (and alpha) linoleic acid – Gratitude** Just as these essential fatty acids are needed for the underlying structure of cells in the body, so too is gratitude required to maintain the underlying structure of your spiritual form. Gratitude helps to construct and make sense out of your life. Count your blessings and express your appreciation to everything and everyone you encounter.

Practical Plan: The enrichment plan ✤

YOU HAVE NOW reached the final month of your Personal Health Action Plan. Before you begin this last phase, I suggest you go right back to the very first activity in your first week of the plan. This activity was a simple goal-setting exercise. You were urged to create goals for yourself – five short-term and five long-term goals. Check out the short-term goals and see how many you can tick off. If you either haven't reached the goals or never performed the exercise, do it now.

It's human nature to tackle a plan or a programme with plenty of enthusiasm at the beginning and then lose interest. Inherent in plans and goals is often the failure factor. It is difficult to sustain many programmes.

If you have followed all parts of the five-month programme so far, keep it up. If you haven't, do not worry. It is a guideline to assist you and not a rigid prescriptive programme. If you have preferred to use this book solely for the gleaning of information, that is fine, too. But I do encourage you to go through the HAP (Health Action Plan) of each of the first six chapters intermittently and check out what areas you think may need attention and just tackle those weak spots or at the very least make sure you have the necessary medical screening done.

If you asked me to choose just *one* tool from the entire action plan to implement into your life, *although I would argue with you to attempt to implement them all in a slow and stepwise fashion*, eventually at your insistence I would relent and offer up **meditation** as *the* one!

You will have noticed that meditation was an exercise from last month's programme (see page 226). The chances are that if you did begin meditating, by now you have stopped.

That's why it is here again! As powerful a practice as it is, so too is meditation difficult to maintain. There is a very good reason for this. You are an active person, interacting all the time with people and the world around you. To sit quietly and 'do nothing' for a short while – no speaking, no eating, no communicating, no reading, no television, no music – just silence and an odd word or mantra to focus on while your head buzzes away with all the things you need to do, and your legs are itching to just jump up and get on with the day – is an activity that soon gets discarded.

Some people find it useful (and more powerful) to meditate in a group. You may want to find a meditation circle or put one together yourself. You could use a guided imagery or meditation CD to begin with.

You now have an understanding of the physical and mental health benefits as well as spiritual benefits of meditation. You also have some practical tips at your disposal from the previous chapter. This week I offer to you a few different meditations to work with.

Before you do any of the following meditations, tell those around you not to disturb you for the next 10 to 20 minutes. Switch off your cell phone and take your phone off the hook.

A. Meditation on your breath

Sit or lie down in a comfortable place and begin by paying attention to your breathing. Follow your breath as it enters and leaves your body. Just observe your breath for a few moments. Then allow your breathing to become slower and deeper, letting your muscles relax with each breath out. As you breathe in, inhale fresh calm energy. As you breathe out, release all your stress and strain. Put one hand on your chest and the other on your abdomen and feel the breath entering and leaving your body.

If most of the movement is in your chest, know you are carrying tension deep within your body. Begin to breathe more and more deeply, feeling the movement within your abdominal muscles.

255

Now stay with this breathing for about 10 minutes and all that you do is concentrate and notice your breath. As soon as you find your mind wandering back to your endless stream of thoughts, just gently go back to paying attention to your breath.

Your breath straddles the border between your physical and spiritual self. Breathing is the only physiological function over which you have control. You can hold your breath. You can slow the pace of your breath. The word for spirit and the word for breath in many languages is one and the same. God literally breathed a breath into the soul of man. You can use this metaphor or visualisation as a meditation, too.

B. Meditation on the breath of Creation

Sit or lie down in a comfortable place and begin by paying attention to your breathing, just as before. Follow your breath as it enters and leaves your body. Just observe your breath for a few moments. Then allow your breathing to become slower and deeper, letting your muscles relax with each breath out. As you breathe in, inhale fresh calm energy. As you breathe out, release all your stress and strain. Now imagine and focus on the breath of God or the Universe surrounding you in a cloud of warmth and light. Feel this breath being transmitted to you and through you. And as you breathe in and out feel this warm, healing, soothing breath becoming one with your breath. Stay with this idea over and over again with each breath you take.

C. Meditation on a word or mantra

Find a comfortable place to sit or lie down. It is preferable to sit upright in a comfortable chair. Close your eyes, uncross your arms and legs and place your hands in your lap or on your legs. You now focus on a single word or image. Some people prefer a 'visual mantra' like a candle or a rose. Most prefer to use a word. If you attend a course of meditation in the school of TM (transcendental meditation) you will be given a word as your mantra, but you can use any mantra. If spiritual awakening is part of your reason for meditating, then it is wonderful to use a word that has a meaning to you. You can use a word such as *God, One, Love* or sentence from a prayer such as *'The Lord is my shepherd'*.

This is one of the most basic forms of meditation. In clinical medical or psychological settings, it is called SCM (Standardised Clinical Meditation) and you simply focus on the word 'ONE'. You simply sit and focus on this word/ mantra for the next 10 to 20 minutes. What will happen is that soon you will be distracted by all the thoughts and ideas spinning through your mind. Don't fight the thoughts. Simply choose to go back to the mantra. The tedious work of mediation is simply returning constantly to the mantra away from your thoughts. Occasionally you may find that for a split second, the very briefest moment, you have neither thought nor mantra – this moment is called transcendence. Experienced meditators experience lengthier periods of transcendence. Do not try too hard. Do not attempt to reach these tracendent moments – the more you try, the less it happens. You need to just do the activity daily and after a few weeks or months and especially years, the benefits become wondrous.

D. Meditation towards a goal

Sit or lie down in a comfortable place and begin by paying attention to your breathing. Follow your breath as it enters and leaves your body. Just observe your breath for a few moments. Then allow your breathing to become slower and deeper, letting your muscles relax with each breath out.

Now focus on just *one* thing you want to do that is not currently part of your life. Choose something specific and imagine in very fine detail what it would look like, feel like, be like to do it. It may be what you are doing right now (meditating), or it may be exercising or painting or dancing or swimming. See yourself in this activity. Feel the movement, feel the emotions. Imagine yourself immersed in the activity.

Now come back to yourself right here at this moment. How are you feeling emotionally and physically? Is there a gap? Are you more tired, less inspired, less calm or fit than you would like to be? Take a few breaths and feel the gap between where you are and where you would like to be. Now imagine yourself beginning right from the place you are. See yourself accomplishing all you wish even though you are tired and distracted. Give yourself permission to begin right from here.

⚹
Week 2:
Fill your spiritual
prescription
⚹

What do you need on your spiritual prescription? Write yourself a script. Take out your Health Action Plan journal and write it out for yourself. First determine what it is you are seeking and what your signs and symptoms are.

Do you have *signs* of 'Spiritual Deficiency Syndrome'?

+ Is something missing in your life?
+ Are you in pain and in need of healing?
+ Are you thirsting for inspiration?
+ Are you craving a sense of community?
+ Are you craving quality time?
+ Are you feeling content and grateful and want to give something back?
+ Are you facing a crisis and need strength?
+ Are you burned out and seriously fatigued?
+ Are you anxious about your loved ones and their safety?

What you require in your script is the spiritual practices, the activities you do to move into deeper relationships with God, yourself and others. You need to choose these activities yourself.

You also need to examine your *symptoms*. You can leave that for next week. You have already begun to nourish, exercise and energise your soul through Week 1's meditation practice. Write your prescription this week. You may choose to just fill it with meditation. You may want to add another spiritual pursuit such as attending a monthly lecture, enrolling in a regular yoga class, making prayer more central in your life. You choose. It is far more beneficial for you to choose only a single spiritual activity and stick with it, rather than shopping around for a whole host of meaningless activities.

𝒥
Week 3:
Nutrients
𝒥

Check out the symptom chart and determine which spiritual vitamins and minerals you need. Obviously they are all beneficial and you would do well to incorporate them all. But focus this week on just three that you most require.

𝒥
Week 4:
Action
𝒥

For almost six months, you have been focused on the suggested activities of the Health Action Plan. You have been encouraged to Take *charge* and empower yourself, Take *care* and embrace yourself and especially Take *action* in what and how you eat, exercise, energise and now enrich yourself. All these actions have been designed to enhance your own health and expand your own life.

This very final action is not about you. It is not about your health. It is not about your personal growth. It is not about your soul. It is about the actions you do for others.

You have garnered from this chapter that the following activities are vitamins for your soul.

But that is not the focus of this very final action. The focus on these **actions** is what you can do for others purely for the sake of creating wellbeing in the world around you. This week pay attention to whatever action you can perform for the benefit of people around you. Extend a helping hand in your office, make that phone call to say hello and I care, visit that friend who lost a loved one recently, use your skills to offer assistance in your neighbourhood, give some charity to a worthy cause. Do something good.

CHAPTER 7

The A-Z of Women's Health Problems

Introduction

This section gives a brief outline of commonly encountered women's health problems, and provides you with updated information as to the prevention and management of these problems. Regardless of which issue or illness pertains to you, the essential task is for you to *take charge* by becoming empowered, to *take excellent care* and responsibility, and then to *take action* – to do all you can to improve your condition and your life. This is by no means an exhaustive list of all medical ailments. Neither is it an intensive medical review of each subject. It does, however, provide a starting point for expanding your knowledge and give you the tools to live a better life.

Ageing

Beginning at about age 30 and moving at a snail's pace, the inevitable process of ageing sets in. Changes begin to occur in your skin's elasticity, your hearing, eyesight, bone density and muscle strength. Your metabolism slows down and physiological function declines. This is manifest in a rising blood pressure, inadequate sugar metabolism (leading to high blood glucose levels and diabetes) and increasing levels of cholesterol. These changes occur extremely slowly and vary significantly from one person to the next.

I believe you can age well and slow the process. Some people have more advanced signs of ageing, not only in the wrinkles on their faces but in their cells and in their biomarkers. These include your blood pressure, cholesterol, blood sugar, metabolic rate, bone density and muscle mass, among others. Genetics do play a role in ageing but a host of other features contribute, too. A most important aspect is how you feel about yourself and your psychological age.

Take charge, take care, take action
Minimise the ageing process by shifting your world view and your perceptions. Age is wisdom, age is experience and age can be beauty and vitality, too. How you see yourself can accelerate or retard this ageing process.

Choose to look after yourself and manage your lifestyle factors. Be sure to keep out of the sun and always use sunscreen to slow down the accelerated ageing changes in your skin. Sun exposure is the number one cause of accelerated ageing to your skin and your cells. Remain active, interested and passionate about people, activities, new ideas and creative endeavours. This keeps you vibrant.

Your nutrition, stress management and exercise play a major part in your ageing. Regular exercise has been shown beyond doubt to retard ageing and is capable of reversing the physiological markers (biomarkers) of ageing. As you age, your nutrition becomes even more important. Make sure you stick to the SELF plan, consuming good-quality proteins, such as salmon; plant-based, best fats e.g. olive oil and avocados; and good quality carbs, like fruits, vegetables and heavy grains. Don't forget your calcium and antioxidant supplements. And do make sure you are managing your stress in any of the different ways that may work for you.

Allergies

Whether or not you'll develop an allergy or not is due to your genetics and environment. A child with one allergic parent has about a 30-50 per cent chance of getting allergies, and if both parents have allergies the chances rise to 60-80 per cent. Exposure to a high level of allergens early on also puts you at increased risk of developing allergic symptoms later.

Your immune system releases histamines and other irritating substances in response to particles like dust, moulds, tree pollen, and animal secretions or hair. Typical allergy symptoms include sneezing, nasal itching and a dripping nose, along with congestion and red, swollen, itchy eyes.

Women rarely develop new allergies after age 30 unless they are exposed to some new allergen such as a pet or a pollen. The good news is that allergies tend to subside at about age 55. That's because your immune system begins to decline, making it less likely to attack an invading mould spore or another allergen.

Take charge, take care, take action
+ A plastic cover over your mattress is a good way of limiting dust mite exposure.
+ Getting rid of dust mites in your bedroom means having a clutter-free room with as little fabric in the form of curtains and banners as possible (preferably simple blinds). It is also preferable to not have carpeting, because vacuuming doesn't clear the dust mites.
+ Remember to change and wash bed linen often.
+ Keep pets out of your room and preferably in a room with no carpets.
+ If you have a fan in your bathroom, turn it on whenever you take a shower or bath. A humid, unventilated bathroom makes mould worse.
+ You may require intermittent treatment with antihistamines, decongestants and even short courses of inhaled or nasal cortisone sprays. Some homeopathic remedies may also be effective.
+ If you know the pollen count is high, or if you're going to visit someone with a cat, take your medication before symptoms begin.
+ Make sure you take the medicine at least 30 minutes to an hour before you're exposed to the allergens.
+ Avoid alcohol. It can worsen symptoms such as congestion, and mixing alcohol with antihistamines can cause serious health problems

Alzheimer's disease
Approximately 8-10 per cent of all those older than 65 and nearly 30-50 per cent of those people older than 85 have Alzheimer's disease. It is a brain condition characterised by progressive intellectual impairment. The exact cause is unknown. At first the only symptom may be mild forgetful-

ness. As the disease progresses, different aspects of brain functioning becomes impaired. A new study (2 September 2004, *Neuron*) suggests that a diet rich in the omega-3 fatty acid called DHA, which is found in salmon, halibut and other cold-water fish, may protect the brain from the damage caused by Alzheimer's.

No treatment is currently available that can stop or cure Alzheimer's, but new medications are available that can improve memory and delay the progression of the illness.

Take charge, take care, take action
Some risk factors for Alzheimer's are beyond your control, such as ageing and a family history. But you may be able to delay or prevent Alzheimer's by adopting the following brain-healthy habits:
✦ High blood pressure and heart disease are both risk factors for Alzheimer's. You can control both by maintaining a healthy body weight, cholesterol level and blood-sugar level.
✦ Regular exercise maintains good blood flow to the brain and lowers your risk of heart disease and stroke.
✦ Participate in activities that stimulate your brain, such as reading, crossword puzzles, studying and attending lectures. Such activities can strengthen brain cells and connections.

Anaemia
Anaemia means a shortage of red blood cells and their contents, called haemoglobin. The symptoms include fatigue, dizziness, light-headedness, fainting, possibly shortness of breath and poor resistance to colds or other infections. It is often difficult to diagnose this common condition. Your doctor will look at your nails and mucous membranes within your eyelid and your tongue to check the colour, but a blood test is required to confirm a diagnosis.

There are many different causes but the commonest is iron-deficiency anaemia. The body needs iron (and plenty of it) to manufacture red blood cells. These red blood cells contain haemoglobin, the protein responsible for transporting oxygen in the blood. With too little iron, you have less haemoglobin, less oxygen and less energy. The predominant cause of iron-deficiency anaemia in women is menstrual blood loss. Women with heavy menstrual flow are more prone to anaemia, because they lose more blood than women with lighter flow. That is why anaemia is more common in premenopausal women when menstrual flow may become heavier. Pregnancy and breastfeeding also drain iron stores, and low dietary intake (or poor iron absorption) also contributes to anemia in women. Other less common causes of anaemia will be excluded by your doctor.

Take charge, take care, take action
✦ Eat iron-rich foods. Although red meats are high in saturated fat and cholesterol, which can contribute to heart disease, they are the best sources of iron, especially liver because it contains the form of iron most completely absorbed by the body. So if you have a tendency to iron-deficiency anaemia or have very heavy periods, eat extra-lean cuts of red meat.
✦ Add folate to your diet. Women with anaemia also tend to run low on folate (one of the B vitamins) and folate deficiency contributes to anaemia. Eat plenty of foods high in folate (such as lentils or spinach) and/or take a supplement of folate (400 micrograms per day).
✦ If your anaemia is more severe, your doctor will most likely prescribe iron supplements of up to 180 mg a day. You are advised against taking iron supplements without a doctor's supervision, because too much iron can be toxic.
✦ Foods high in vitamin C enhance iron absorption. Take your supplement with a glass of orange or cranberry juice. Other good food sources of vitamin C include guavas, kiwi fruit, red peppers, pawpaws and strawberries.
✦ Do not expect an improvement overnight. You should take your supplements for at least six months but a year is best. You may feel better in a few weeks because your blood level of iron is restored. However, it takes longer to restore the iron stores in your bone marrow. So keep on with the supplement for as long as advised by your doctor.

Anxiety

Generalised anxiety disorder is a mental illness that causes a person to have persistent nagging feelings of worry. These feelings are either unusually intense, or out of proportion to the real troubles and dangers of the person's everyday life. Anxiety can range from a mild irritability and gnawing pit in your stomach, right through to a severe generalised anxiety disorder with depression. There is often no clear dividing line between normal worry and generalised anxiety disorder. People with the disorder typically experience excessive worry almost every day, for a period of six months or more. In some cases, a person with generalised anxiety disorder finds it hard to remember a time when she was not always worrying.

Anxiety can keep you up at night, make you irritable and undermine your ability to concentrate. And this constant anxious feeling keeps your adrenalin pumping, your heart racing and your palms sweating. Anxiety is often confused with fear. With fear you generally know what's frightening you, whereas with anxiety it is impossible to determine the cause of the worry. People with generalised anxiety disorder have a variety of noticeable physical symptoms, and often first seek treatment with a medical doctor or specialist – most often a cardiologist as they complain of palpitations and chest pain.

Take charge, take care, take action

If you feel anxious most of the time, you should seek help. A few sessions with a psychologist may give an indication of the severity of the anxiety. A number of psychotherapy techniques may be very helpful in treating your anxiety, such as:

✦ Meditation (see pages 228 and 257) promotes a calmness that eases anxious feelings and offers a sense of control. Many studies have demonstrated that those who embarked on a daily meditation practice were considerably less anxious after a few weeks.
✦ Exercise can have the same calming effect as meditation, particularly if it's something repetitive like running or swimming laps.
✦ Breathing slowly and deeply can have a calming effect, too.
✦ If the anxiety is seriously interfering with your ability to work or

establish and maintain relationships, or if you are always on edge or expecting the worst, you need to see a professional. Medication may be needed. Certain antidepressants (SSRIs – selective serotonin reuptake inhibitors) and anxiolytics are very effective in treating anxiety disorders. With appropriate treatment, more than 50 per cent of patients improve within three to six weeks of starting medication.

Panic disorder

Panic disorder is a type of anxiety disorder in which a person experiences panic attacks. These attacks are repeated, unexpected episodes of intense fear and anxiety, along with physical symptoms linked to the body's normal response to danger. When you experience true danger (such as a confrontation with a hijacker armed with a gun), your body automatically releases adrenalin and goes into a 'fight or flight' reaction. You will become intensely fearful and highly alert. Your heart rate increases and you start to feel a pounding in your chest, blood rushes to your arms and leg muscles, causing a trembling or tingling feeling, and your palms becomes sweaty.

In a panic attack these changes occur without any real danger. At the height of the attack a person may feel that she is going to die or have a heart attack. Some people may experience several panic attacks each day, while others may not have any attacks for several weeks or months. Since panic attacks typically occur without warning, sufferers often live in constant fear, anticipating an attack at any moment.

A panic attack is having at least four of the following symptoms:

✦ Palpitations, pounding heart or a rapid pulse
✦ Sweating
✦ Trembling or shaking
✦ Breathing problems, especially shortness of breath or a feeling of choking
✦ Chest pain or chest discomfort
✦ Abdominal discomfort, upset stomach or nausea
✦ Feeling faint, dizzy, light-headed or unsteady on your feet
✦ A feeling that things around you are strange and you are detached from yourself

✦ Fear that you will lose control or 'go crazy'
✦ Fear of dying
✦ Numbness or tingling in your arms, legs or other parts of your body
✦ Chills or hot flushes

Take charge, take care, take action
You may be able to reduce panic attacks by cutting down on caffeine, alcohol or other substances that might trigger your symptoms, but you will probably still require medication which will give long-term relief from the attacks. Several treatment options include the use of benzodiazepines which bring quick relief from the intense fear and anxiety that accompany panic attacks. They may be used only during the first weeks of treatment while you are waiting for other medications such as antidepressants, to start working. Antidepressants are the main treatment for panic attacks, especially when they keep occurring or if you also have depression.

✦ Non-medical therapies include cognitive and behaviour therapy. For many patients, the most effective approach is a combination of one or more medications, plus some form of cognitive or behaviour therapy. With appropriate treatment, the prognosis is good.

✦ Several European countries have approved the use of a herbal preparation called Kava kava in the treatment of mild anxiety. Kavain/Kava kava was compared to standard benzodiazepines and proved as effective (as the standard medication) for *mild* anxiety with none of the addictive side effects.

At recommended levels kava extracts have shown no side effects in otherwise healthy individuals, but side effects may develop at high dosages. Kava kava should not be used in people with Parkinson's disease.

✦ Remedies for mild anxiety include Bach flower therapies such as Rescue remedy, as well as homeopathic preparations. If you suffer from a *severe* generalised anxiety or panic disorder, you will need appropriate allopathic medication as alternate remedies are unlikely to be effective.

Arthritis

The two most common forms of arthritis are osteoarthritis and rheumatoid arthritis. The 'wear-and-tear' arthritis, called osteoarthritis (or OA), is a degenerative joint disease that usually affects people over the age of 45. Rheumatoid arthritis is an inflammatory autoimmune disease that can occur in people from as young as 30, but occurs most frequently between the ages of 40 and 60. An autoimmune condition means that your body erroneously detects normal structures within your body as foreign and creates antibodies against these structures. So antibodies (the same immune substances that fight infections) create a reaction against certain tissue, and inflammation occurs in these tissues. Rheumatoid arthritis is two to three times more common in women than men. It is more widespread than osteoarthritis and it can affect every tissue in the body.

Take charge, take care, take action

✦ The key to living well with any form of arthritis is to get an early, accurate diagnosis. Tell your doctor if you experience any of the following:

  ⭒ Pain, stiffness, warmth, redness or swelling at the joints, wrists, fingers, neck, shoulders, elbows, hips, knees, ankles and feet

  ⭒ Pain or stiffness in the morning, lasting more than 30 minutes

  ⭒ Fatigue

  ⭒ Occasional fever.

✦ To manage your arthritis well, some type of exercise is needed to strengthen the muscles that support the joints. For example, if arthritis affects your knees, walking up or down stairs may be really painful. If you strengthen your knee muscles, then those stairs won't be so hard to manage. If you have access to a pool, especially a heated pool, use it often! Water exercise benefits almost everyone with arthritis. A good form of exercise is riding a stationary bike. Cycling for 20-30 minutes three times a week has been shown to improve function and reduces pain.

✦ Heat and cold therapy may ease pain. For relief of pain, ice packs alternating with heat packs are very effective.

✦ Your doctor will suggest the best form of medication to reduce inflammation and pain. Make sure you review your medication programme from time to time. Often an arthritis sufferer is prescribed more and more medications by different physicians and no-one says *'Let's stop right here and review what is absolutely necessary'.* You as an empowered patient may need to be the one to do that!

✦ Support swollen joints. Splinting a joint with a simple wrist splint can ease pain.

✦ You may find that you wake up with stiff, swollen hands. This is because body fluids during the night may swell in fingers that may already be swollen. To reduce swelling and pain, consider wearing a snug pair of stretch gloves while you sleep.

✦ Some kinds of arthritis cause vaginal dryness and sex therefore can be painful. If no one has told you about this, be reassured that you can do something. Get an over-the-counter vaginal moisturiser and use it regularly, as directed.

Asthma

Asthma is a chronic disease and you may need long-term treatment. In most cases, good control can be achieved and there is little reason why asthma sufferers cannot lead a perfectly normal life. Just what causes asthma remains something of a mystery. There certainly may be a family history of asthma and allergies, but not in all cases. Unfortunately, this condition often goes undiagnosed and untreated in many people. You can develop it at any age. Many women are diagnosed between the ages of 45 and 55.

According to some doctors, asthma is the great hidden women's issue. Research in the United States shows that 75 per cent of adults hospitalised with asthma attacks are women. Other researchers have found that since 1982, the asthma rate among adult women has almost doubled. What makes women more vulnerable? Studies have revealed that there may be a hormonal link because many of the attacks occur just prior to and during menstruation (Dr Emil Skobeloff, Prof Allegheny University, Philadelphia). The asthma-menstrual cycle link may be related to changes in women's oestrogen levels. Your asthma may feel better during your pregnancy but it not advisable to stop your medication as you may develop an acute attack. Please discuss your medication with your doctor.

The symptoms of asthma include wheezing, coughing and a tight chest which may be worsened with exercise. But having asthma need not hinder your performance or prevent you from exercising. Use your inhaler prior to exercising but active asthmatics, particularly those who are competitive sportspeople, report that they feel more in control of their asthma when they're fit.

Many women look for alternative ways to treat asthma with homeopathic and natural approaches. Homoeopathic medicines may help to boost your immune system but are not recommended as the sole treatment for asthma.

Take charge, take care, take action

✦ Take your medication regularly. These may be a combination of inhaled bronchodilators, inhaled corticosteroids, cromolyns or leukotriene inhibitors. By neglecting your treatment, you may trigger an acute attack or go on to cause long-term damage to your lungs.

✦ Use a peak flow meter regularly to monitor day-to-day variations in your breathing and lung capacity and to identify if your condition is worsening.

✦ Identify what triggers your attacks and, where possible, remove them from your life. Common triggers include house dust mites, cockroaches, pollens, outdoor moulds and tobacco smoke.

✦ You may also need to make some lifestyle changes that will help keep you on top form. Smoking is absolutely out of the question. Moderate exercise is good for your asthma.

✦ Rush to your closest hospital if:

   ★ Your symptoms get worse even after taking extra medication.

   ★ You're having a hard time breathing (or your peak flow has dropped below 50 per cent).

   ★ You're struggling to walk or talk.

   ★ Your lips and fingernails are turning blue-grey.

Bladder problems

The two most common bladder troubles are urinary tract infections (UTIs) and bladder incontinence. Incontinence is not only a nuisance for elderly women, there are causes for incontinence in younger women as well.

1. Bladder infections (urinary tract infections)

These are extremely common in women. Ten to twenty per cent of all women have some urinary tract discomfort or infection at least once a year. Almost 50 per cent of women have had a urinary tract infection (UTI) in the past 10 years. Recurrent bladder infections can be a significant problem and can even affect the kidneys, causing scarring and damage.

Your bladder and the urine it holds are normally free from bacteria and other organisms. A urinary tract infection occurs when organisms are introduced into the bladder. Bacteria from the skin may enter through your urethra, the tube that carries urine from the bladder to the outside of the body. UTIs are much less common in males, the reason being that women have a shorter urethra which allows easier access for these bacteria.

The most common symptoms of a UTI are frequent urination, burning on urination and urgency or the need to empty the bladder immediately. UTIs may also cause lower abdominal pain, a bloody, pink or cloudy urine, nausea and vomiting, strong smelling urine, fever and chills and burning on intercourse. The most common cause of a UTI is a bacteria called E. coli. These bacteria are normally present in the bowel and faeces. They can be introduced into the bladder by sexual activity. When older people get a UTI, it is often associated with confusion and mental changes.

Take charge, take care, take action
To prevent infections:
+ Always empty your bladder completely.
+ Always wipe from front to back after a bowel movement.
+ Avoid chemicals that may irritate the urethra, such as strong soaps.
+ Avoid going for long periods without emptying the bladder.
+ Try to empty your bladder following intercourse to flush out any possible bacteria that were introduced during sexual activity.

Once your doctor has diagnosed a UTI you will need an antibiotic. Without adequate treatment, the infection may spread to your kidneys. Urinary symptoms usually clear up within the first three days of antibiotic therapy. If symptoms persist or worsen, contact your doctor.

2. Incontinence

Urinary incontinence is a condition where you unintentionally leak urine, and is very common in women. A common cause of incontinence, especially in older women, is a vaginal prolapse. The main symptom is urinary incontinence, but you may also experience some anal incontinence and pain on intercourse. The vaginal prolapse generally progresses slowly but becomes most uncomfortable and embarrassing and interferes with your daily life. You must have it assessed and carefully consider the different forms of treatment. The different types of incontinence are:

Stress incontinence: Due to weakness in pelvic floor muscles and may be caused by childbirth or pelvic surgery. You may leak urine when you exercise, cough, sneeze, laugh, lift or put pressure on your abdomen

Urge incontinence: This is the most common form of incontinence. It may cause you to lose urine as soon as you have the urge to go to the bathroom or even when you drink a small amount of liquid. It also may result in frequent urination (every half-hour, for example) or bedwetting.

Overflow incontinence: With overflow incontinence you may feel as though you never completely empty your bladder. You pass only a small amount of urine and feel your bladder is still full. Or you may feel as if you have to empty your bladder but can't.

Transient incontinence: This is temporary incontinence that occurs due to certain conditions, including urinary tract infections, the use of some medications and restricted mobility.

An accurate diagnosis is essential. Your doctor needs to take a detailed history in order to categorise the problem. Additional tests may be required to obtain the correct diagnosis. These tests include a urine specimen, ultrasound, cystoscopy and cystometry. Not all tests need to be performed in every patient; the urine specimen and cystometry are the more important ones.

Surgery is only helpful in stress incontinence, which is why the correct diagnosis is important.

Take charge, take care, take action

Once you have a diagnosis there is much you can do. Discuss the options with your doctor once you have been fully assessed.

+ Less weight means less strain on the bladder. This may not resolve the problem completely but it will be extremely helpful.
+ Pelvic floor exercises are extremely important. If you have ever attended labour classes you will remember these as Kegel exercises. Making the muscles of the pelvis stronger will enable the bladder to better withstand pressure during straining (e.g. coughing, laughing, sneezing). Many physiotherapists are able to train you in these exercises.
+ Oestrogens are important in maintaining healthy pelvic tissues. After menopause, when your ovaries stop producing oestrogen, the pelvic tissues may become weaker leading to stress incontinence. Hormone replacement may be prescribed in the form of cream, patches or tablets to strengthen the pelvic tissues.
+ Control of the bladder may be achieved by voiding on command, rather than when you feel the urge. This can be very effective in controlling urge incontinence.
+ Make sure if you have diabetes, that your sugar is well controlled.
+ Limiting fluid intake before setting out on long journeys, going out or at night can help reduce incontinence by keeping the bladder relatively empty.
+ Avoid caffeine in tea, coffee and cola drinks as this can make urge incontinence worse and cause an increased production of urine.
+ Avoid acidic foods such as tomatoes and lemon. Artificial sweeteners also seem to affect the bladder and worsen urgency.

Blood pressure (Hypertension)

Your blood pressure is a measure of the pressure as your blood is pumped out of your heart. It is extremely important to have your blood pressure checked regularly, especially as you get older. High blood pressure, or hypertension, can cause damage to your heart and is a risk factor for developing a stroke. Even if extremely high, it may cause no symptoms. It is for this reason that high blood pressure is called the silent killer.

People often complain of low blood pressure. This is not a problem at all and is generally a healthy sign. If it is very low, you may feel dizzy, especially in hot weather. You would do well to increase your fluid intake.

Take charge, take care, take action

✦ Have your blood pressure checked to establish a baseline reading. This is an easy, non-invasive investigation that can be done by your doctor or clinic nurse. It is important to have at least two or three readings on separate occasions before a diagnosis is made. You should attempt to get it checked every second year and then preferably yearly beyond age 45. High blood pressure is best managed with a combination of lifestyle changes, such as weight loss, exercise and diet (salt restriction) and effective medication.

✦ Your BP should be regularly checked by your doctor, preferably always the same doctor, to ensure that it is well controlled. High blood pressure, if untreated, can eventually lead to heart disease and stroke.

✦ If you are overweight, your blood pressure will most certainly drop when you shed those extra kilos.

✦ Regular moderate exercise can help reduce existing hypertension and also prevent you ever developing high blood pressure, even if you have a genetic predisposition.

✦ Eating a low-salt diet can protect the arteries from stiffening.

✦ Very recent research has demonstrated that a folate supplement – folic acid, already known for its power to prevent birth defects – also appears to reduce the risk of high blood pressure for women both young and old. (Dr John Forman, October 2004 American Heart Association conference, Chicago.)

Breast cancer

Breast cancer is the leading cause of cancer deaths in women globally. South African women are under the false impression that breast cancer is a white woman's disease and that it affects only older women. It's incidence is highest in Indian women and dramatically on the increase in black women and very young women, too.

Take charge, take care, take action

Screening for breast cancer is essential. If breast cancer is detected before it has spread to tissues outside the breast, the survival rate is more than 95 percent. It is a remarkably asymptomatic condition in many patients and if it is not detected by breast self-examination as a lump or with a routine mammogram, it can remain undetected until it has reached an advanced stage.

The mainstay of early detection includes BSE (breast self-examination) and mammograms. It is also important to be examined at least once a year by your doctor or gynaecologist. Many mammography centres now perform an ultrasound (sonar) of your breast as well as the mammogram, as it has been shown to increase the pick up rate of early cancer.

1. Breast self-examination

You should check your breasts every month for lumps. By checking regularly you get to know the normal structure of your breast and can identify a lump at a very early stage. The earlier the breast cancer is detected, the better your long-term outcome. The best time to check is a week after the onset of your period. The generalised lumpiness of your breasts just prior and during your period may interfere with your self-examination. If you are no longer menstruating then choose a date each month to check yourself.

2. Mammogram

A mammogram is a low-dose breast x-ray that can detect breast cancer even before a lump is felt. X-ray pictures are taken of the top and sides of your breasts, which are compressed between x-ray plates. The compression causes little or no discomfort in most women and does not damage breast tissue. A baseline mammogram at the age of 40 is highly recommended and then should be performed at least every two years, preferably every year.

If any abnormality is detected, please remember that 80 per cent of breast lumps are benign (non-cancerous). If an abnormality or lump is found, you may need another type of test (an ultrasound) or your doctor may need to draw fluid from the lump (aspiration) or remove a section of the lump (biopsy) in order to make a diagnosis. If advised by a doctor, women at higher risk may undergo mammograms more often and at an earlier age than recommended for the general population.

Cancer

The advent of a cancer in your life may be fraught with unpleasant therapies, fear and uncertainty. But there are many types of curable cancer, especially if detected early. Much can be done to empower yourself once the reality of the shock has passed. The most important thing is to arm yourself with as much knowledge as you feel comfortable with and to participate as much as possible in the decision-making regarding your treatment plan. It is a good idea to involve your partner, a family member or friend who will be available to support you through this.

Take charge, take care, take action
Always be vigilant about strange symptoms that persist and do not resolve within a short period of time. Obviously you need not overreact to every new symptom; the overwhelming majority of physical symptoms are due to common, unimportant ailments. But if any of these persist, have them checked with your family doctor or local clinic. *Do not ignore the following changes:*

✦ A lump anywhere in your body that persists or grows larger.
✦ A growth or lump in your neck.
✦ Any postmenopausal vaginal bleeding if you are not on HRT.
✦ A skin mole or spot which enlarges, itches or bleeds.
✦ A chronic cough or a new cough productive of blood.

✦ A huge loss of weight (without dieting).
✦ A loss of appetite for an extended period of time.

Breast cancer

The most common cancer in South African women is breast cancer (see page 276).

Cancer of the cervix

This is extremely widespread in South Africa although on the decrease in the rest of the world. It is one of the few preventable cancers because it is so easy to diagnose the premalignant stage with a simple Pap smear. Unfortunately, women are still dying from this preventable cancer. Be proactive about this yearly investigation (see Pap smears, page 314).

Uterine cancer

Uterine cancer accounts for about 13 per cent of all cancers in women. There are two distinct points within the uterus where cancer may originate: the endometrium and the uterine wall.

1. **Endometrial cancer:** The endometrium is the inner lining of the uterus where the most common type of uterine cancer occurs. Women between the ages of 50 and 65 are most affected. High levels of estrogen, while not a danger by itself, poses a risk for endometrial cancer when not offset by the hormone progesterone. Since progesterone levels decrease after menopause, postmenopausal women are particularly at risk. Other conditions associated with a high level of unopposed estrogen include obesity, and long-term oestrogen replacement therapy. Any vaginal bleeding after menopause must be checked out. If you are taking hormone replacement therapy and experience any bleeding other than at the expected time, please contact your doctor who will do a check of your endometrium.

2. **Uterine sarcoma:** The uterine wall consists of connective tissues, such as muscle, fat, bone and fibrous tissue. Cancers beginning in this type of tissue are called sarcomas. Uterine sarcoma is rare.

Colorectal cancer

Cancer of the colon or rectum is a very common cancer killer in women. It is a condition that can be detected early, long before it becomes symptomatic. Colorectal tumours begin as polyps (small growths) on the inside of the large intestine. Polyps that aren't removed can eventually become cancerous, penetrate through the wall of the colon or rectum, and spread to other areas. The older you get, the more likely you are to develop colorectal cancer.

The best defense against colorectal cancer is regular screening. Screening tests are designed to find benign polyps (precancerous growths) that can be removed before they become cancerous (malignant) and catch cancer at an early stage when it is easier to cure. Unfortunately cancer of the colon is usually only discovered at a much later stage when treatment is not effective. It is recommended that all adults begin screening for colorectal cancer at age 50. People at higher risk should begin screening earlier. Recommended screening methods include:

1. **Rectal examination:** performed by your doctor, baseline at at age 40, then yearly after 50. This should not be used as the only screening method.

2. **Faecal occult blood** is a simple, cheap and absolutely painless test. It should be performed after age 45 years. You need to ask your clinic or doctor to give you a specimen bottle in which to place a stool sample, which is then tested in the laboratory for blood (which cannot be seen with the naked eye). If this early change is present, further investigation (e.g. colonoscopy) and highly effective treatment is available.

3. **Colonoscopy:** Many doctors recommend this as a screening procedure for all people over age 50 and earlier if you have a family history. Colonoscopy should then be performed every five to 10 years.

Factors that increase the risk of developing colorectal cancer include family history, inflammatory bowel disease (e.g. Crohn's or ulcerative colitis), poor diet (low in fibre and high in fat), and a sedentary lifestyle.

If you experience symptoms such as a change in bowel habits e.g. a recent onset of diarrhoea or constipation, blood in the stool (bright red,

black or very dark), a feeling that the bowel does not empty completely
and weight loss without dieting, please consult your doctor.

Complementary therapy for cancer?
I do encourage you to use complementary techniques to optimise your
condition and augment your healing. But always consult your doctor first,
and even if he or she does not believe in the therapy, just make sure that
no harm can be done. These therapies may give you support, comfort or
may aid your healing. You may choose to learn meditation, practise
guided imagery, relaxation techniques, acupuncture, reflexology, Ayur-
vedic or Chinese medicine or follow a sound nutritional plan. Steer clear
of any practitioner who tells you there is only one way to heal from cancer and that is with his/her therapy, or anyone who advises you to forego
the treatment advised by your doctor. This is extremely dangerous.

You can choose to become empowered and active in your cancer
therapy. Ensure that you receive optimal medical therapy first, with excellent emotional support including a good doctor-patient relationship (if
possible). Implementing mind-body techniques and living with a sense
of faith have also been shown to support the healing process.

Cholesterol
Cholesterol is one of a large and important class of molecules called
lipids, which is the scientific jargon for fats. This fatty substance, present
normally in the bloodstream and in all your tissues and cells, is absolutely
necessary for human life. Lipids and cholesterol form an important function as part of the architecture of cell wall and cellular structures.
Cholesterol is manufactured in your liver as well as consumed in your
diet. The popular view that cholesterol is the root cause of all heart disease is overly simplistic. You need to understand the role of fats as well as
the many risk factors for heart disease.

Take charge, take care, take action
Check out your baseline cholesterol and if it is normal, you only need to
test it every five years. A cholesterol check involves a simple blood test at

Table 1

Description	Cholesterol levels	Take action
Desirable	Total cholesterol below 5 mmol/l; HDL more than 0,9 mmol/l	☆ Retest in five years; ☆ Further evaluation if smoking, hypertension
Borderline to high	Total cholesterol 5-7,5 mmol/l	☆ Follow-up visits every 6-12 months. Discuss with doctor whether lipid lowering drugs are needed or not; ☆ Change lifestyle: exercise, low-fat diet and stop smoking; ☆ Risk for heart disease increases with smoking, hypertension and other risk factors
High risk	Total cholesterol 7,5 or higher.	☆ Detailed assessment of blood tests should be done; ☆ Drug therapy should be considered, plus lifestyle changes; ☆ Essential to lower cholesterol levels; ☆ Check out additional risk factors

your local clinic, hospital and at many pharmacies, often at no cost. This approximate testing may suggest a problem but is frequently inaccurate, so a follow-up full cholesterol or what is called a lipogram may need to be performed. There are 4.5 million South Africans with raised cholesterol levels. A high blood cholesterol is a known risk factor for heart disease, so lowering your cholesterol can save your life.

The good news is that often just altering your diet can do the trick. Switch from high-fat foods (eggs, fatty red meats, palm or coconut oil, dairy products made with whole milk) to fresh fruits and vegetables, wholegrain breads and cereals and low-fat dairy products. If diet alone does not lower your levels sufficiently, you may need to be on cholesterol-lowering medication to reduce your risk of heart and other vascular disease. Exercise can also help lower your risk for the disease.

Atherosclerosis, also known as arteriosclerosis or 'hardening of the arteries', is a disease process that causes narrowing of the arteries and thickening of the artery walls. It occurs to some extent as people get older, but more rapidly in some individuals for reasons which are largely preventable. It is caused by build-up of deposits such as cholesterol in the blood. This can result in serious medical problems such as a heart attack or stroke. There is no cure for atherosclerosis though surgery and related procedures can relieve blockages in specific places. The major treatment goal is to reduce progression and complications when atherosclerosis has already presented clinically. However, it is better to prevent the development of significant disease in the first place.

Understanding the cholesterol numbers
Once your cholesterol has been tested, your doctor will also look at other lipid (fat) levels from your blood profile to decide what is the best approach. Here is a basic guide to understand your levels:

Contraception
Your choice of contraception is a very personal one. It depends on your stage in life, your relationship and any medical or gynaecological problems. Because these and other factors need to be taken into account you need to be extremely knowledgeable about the options.

Ideally you should discuss this subject openly with your partner and the responsibility for contraception should be a shared one. Unfortunately, this does not often happen and you as a woman therefore need to be vigilant about taking charge.

The best options available for young women include condoms or the oral contraceptive (OC) pill. If you are in a marriage or a stable monogamous relationship with one sexual partner, you have the choice of the OC pill or condoms as well as other options such as the intra-uterine contraceptive device (IUCD, commonly known as the loop) and male vasectomy or tubal ligation (if you have completed your family). As you get into your forties, if you have many cardiovascular risk factors or if you have been on the oral contraceptive pill for many years, you may need to change your form of contraception. (See *Table 2 Contraception choices* on pages 284-285)

Depression

Life is full of emotional ups and downs. But when your 'down' times are long lasting or interfere with your ability to function, you may be suffering from a common problem that needs attention – depression. Clinical depression affects your physical wellbeing, commonly resulting in sleep problems, chronic fatigue and loss of appetite. It affects your mood, with feelings of sadness, emptiness, hopelessness, irritability, social withdrawal and no desire to engage in pleasurable activities, especially a loss of your libido. It affects the way you think and interferes with your concentration and decision making. Research indicates that more than two-thirds of people with depression do not get the help they need. Proper treatment would alleviate the symptoms in over 85 per cent of the cases. Yet, because depression is often unrecognised or is seen as a weakness, you may continue to suffer needlessly. There is absolutely no shame in becoming depressed. It is not your fault. In the same way as anaemia or high blood pressure needs attention, so does depression.

Women are almost twice as likely as men to experience depression. This two-to-one ratio exists regardless of racial and ethnic background or economic status. The reasons for this are not fully understood. Hormones do play a role but this does not explain everything.

Without treatment, symptoms can last for weeks, months or years. However, good treatment in the form of antidepressants and/or psychotherapy can help most people. Treatment will not eliminate life's inevitable stresses and ups and downs, but it can greatly enhance your ability to manage such challenges and lead to greater quality of life.

Take charge, take care, take action

If you experience several of these symptoms or some of the symptoms persist for more than two weeks, or if they interfere with your work and your family life, you should talk to a psychologist or your family doctor:

✦ A continuous sad, anxious or 'empty' mood
✦ Loss of interest or pleasure in your usual activities, including sex
✦ Sleeping too much or too little, early morning waking (this is usually one of the first signs)

Table 2: Contraception choices

Type	Advantages
Condoms	☆ Easy to use ☆ Added protection against HIV and STIs (sexually transmitted infections)
Combined oral contraceptive pill	☆ Highly effective contraception Maintains regulare cycles
Progesterone-only pill (mini-pill)	Good form of contraception whilst breastfeeding
IUD (loop)	☆ Once in, you need not worry about it for up to 5 years
Femdom: female condom	Female in control of contraception and STI prevention
Depo Provera injection	☆ Require shot every 8-12 weeks ☆ Cheap
Tubal ligation	If you're 100% sure you don't want more children
Vasectomy	
Spermicides	
Morning-after pill (emergency contaception)	High dose of progestogen taken in 2 doses 12 hours apart as soon as possible after unprotected sex – maximum period of 72 hrs

✦ Restlessness, irritability or excessive crying
✦ Feelings of guilt, worthlessness, helplessness and hopelessness
✦ Appetite and/or weight loss or overeating and weight gain
✦ Decreased energy, fatigue, feeling 'slowed down'
✦ Thoughts of death or suicide

Disadvantages	Protection	Side effects
★ Possible 3% pregnancy chance; ★ Less sexual satisfaction	96% pregnancy protection	Extremely rare allergy to the latex/rubber
★ Need good compliance; ★ Skipping pills will lead to conception	High rate of protection 99.6%	★ Possible bloating, nausea, irritability in few individuals; ★ Decreased libido common
Decreased libido	Lower rate of protection (98%) than combined. But effective together with breastfeeding	★ Fluid retention; ★ Headaches
If multiple partners, high incidence of infection	96% without added progesterone. 99% with added hormone (Mirena)	Intermittent spotting
★ Tricky to insert; – Less effective than condom against STIs and HIV; ★ 'Noisy' during intercourse;	98% effective	
★ Can take 6-12 months to wear off	99% effective	★ Irregular bleeding ★ Weight gain ★ Depression
Not generally reversible	Most effective almost 100%	
Seldom reversible		
Not very effective		
For EMERGENCY only	80% effective	

- ✦ Difficulty concentrating, remembering or making decisions
- ✦ Persistent physical symptoms that do not respond to treatment, such as headaches, digestive disorders, or chronic pain.

Some people use alcohol, pain medication or drugs to cope with these symptoms. While such drugs may provide temporary relief, they will eventually complicate your depressive disorder and its treatment, and can lead to drug dependence and other major problems. If you use an excessive number of pain killers or sleeping pills and think that you need them for bad headaches or backaches, consult your doctor.

Risks for depression

Many factors unique to women may play a role in the development of depression:

Adolescence: Studies show that the higher incidence of depression in females begins in adolescence, but do not overanalyse your teen daughter as there are many 'normal' behavioural changes that may resemble depression.

Stress: Stress can contribute to depression in many women. These stresses include major responsibilities at home and work, single parenthood, and caring for children and ageing parents.

Hormonal and reproductive stages: Researchers have confirmed that hormones do have an effect on your brain chemistry.

Post-partum depression: This has become an increasingly common condition. Following childbirth almost all women experience a normal moodiness called transient 'blues' or 'day three' weepiness. A post-partum depression is different and may occur any time from immediately after the delivery for up to a year or more after the birth of your child. It may be a severe, incapacitating depression, disturbing for both the woman and her partner. She feels helpless and miserable and is often unable to take care of her new infant. This compounds the depression with feelings of terrible guilt. Seek help immediately, even if you think there is only a slight possibility of this depression. Treatment is extremely effective.

Personality types: Studies show that women with certain characteristics, such as pessimistic thinking, low self-esteem, a sense of having little control over life events, and proneness to excessive worrying, are more likely to develop depression.

Abuse: Studies show that women who have been molested as children are more likely to have clinical depression at some time in their lives than those with no such history. In addition, several studies show a higher incidence of depression among women who were raped as adults.

Poverty: Some researchers are exploring the possibility that poverty is one of the 'pathways to depression'. Low economic status brings with it many stresses but research has not yet established whether depression is more prevalent among those facing the stressors of poverty or not.

Ageing and menopause: Depression should not be dismissed as a normal consequence of ageing. It should be properly evaluated and treated effectively. Depression at menopause used to be considered a unique illness known as 'involutional melancholia'. Research has shown, however, that depressive illnesses are no different, and no more likely to occur at menopause than at other ages.

Treatment for depression

Even severe depression can be highly responsive to treatment. The most commonly used treatments for depression are psychotherapy and antidepressant medication, or a combination of the two.

Psychotherapy is highly effective and appropriate in mild to moderate depression. But in severe or incapacitating depression, in addition to psychotherapy, medication is recommended. In combined treatment, medication can relieve physical symptoms quickly, while psychotherapy allows you to learn more effective ways of handling your problems.

Medication: The advent of newer effective antidepressants in the recent past have opened up possibilities for achieving wellbeing and healing for many sufferers. But there is no doubt that significant controversy about the use of antidepressants abounds. Contrary to popular belief antidepressant medications are not habit-forming. To be effective, medications must be taken for about four to six months and preferably up to a year, carefully following your doctor's instructions. Medications must be monitored to ensure the most effective dosage and to minimise side effects. Please be assertive with your doctor to provide you with as much information as possible about side effects as well as potential drug interactions with any other medication that you may be taking.

If you are suffering from a significant depression, you need to get all the help possible. If that involves taking medication, trust that you need it and it will assist your recovery. But you do need to be aware of the side effects which may include agitation (only at the beginning of therapy), insomnia, weight gain or weight loss, emotional numbness and most commonly a loss of libido. Developing a good rapport with your doctor and therapist is essential to your recovery.

Diabetes

Insulin is a hormone that controls the provision of blood sugar (glucose) to the tissues of your body where it's used for energy. Diabetes is a metabolic disease that affects your body's ability to make or respond to insulin. Type 1, or insulin-dependent diabetes, is an inherited disease that affects your pancreas, destroying its ability to make insulin. Type 1 diabetes usually occurs during childhood or adolescence.

Ninety per cent of people with diabetes have type 2 (or non-insulin-dependent) diabetes. In this type, your body cannot use the insulin properly. Type 2 diabetes usually occurs after age 30.

Take charge, take care, take action

✦ If you have a family history of diabetes, watch out for any signs or symptoms. Ensure that you do not gain excessive weight and that your diet is wholesome and nutritious. See your doctor if you have any of the following symptoms for more than a week.
   ☆ Excessive thirst
   ☆ Markedly increased appetite

* Very frequent urination
* Dizziness
* Weight loss (without dieting)
* Recurrent urinary tract infections
* Dry mouth
* Vomiting, diarrhoea
* Blurred vision

◆ See your doctor if you have diabetes and you're pregnant or thinking of starting a family. Women with poorly controlled diabetes have a higher risk of complicated pregnancies that could affect mother and baby.

◆ If you are diabetic, make sure you are completely in control of your condition.

◆ You need to ensure that you are well monitored, that your blood sugar levels are stable and that you attempt to prevent the onset of organ damage. Keep a close check (with your doctor's assistance) of your blood pressure, your eyes, your kidney function and your heart. Women with diabetes are also prone to problems with circulation or loss of feeling in their feet. So inspect your feet for red, cracked skin, infections and calluses or blisters. And see your doctor if you see signs of infection.

Untreated, even minor cuts or infections can lead to serious medical problems.

◆ Exercise actually makes your muscles more sensitive to insulin, which improves the way your body metabolises sugar. Exercise will also help keep your weight under control and will be reducing your risk of heart disease, a special concern for people with diabetes.

◆ Four out of five women with type 2 diabetes are overweight, and you will certainly improve control of the diabetes or reduce your medication if you lose weight. Reduce your calorie intake and eat the best quality low-fat diet possible. Only eat a moderate amount of carbohydrates and only low GI (Glycaemic Index) carbs (see page 103). Add fibre to your diet in the form of pulses, grains, fresh fruits and vegetables, as it may help regulate blood sugar.

✦ Not everyone agrees with this but tests show that people with diabetes may have lower blood levels of chromium. Your body may need chromium to be able to respond to insulin. It is sometimes difficult to get sufficient amounts of chromium from food, so look for a multivitamin that supplies the recommended amount for chromium (50 to 200 micrograms daily).

✦ Although changes in diet, exercise and the other self-care strategies are important, you should be under high-quality medical supervision.

Eating disorders

Real eating disorders are amongst the most deadly of all mental illnesses, and among the most difficult to treat. They involve serious disturbances in eating behaviour, such as extreme and unhealthy reduction of food intake or severe overeating, as well as feelings of distress or extreme concern about body shape or weight.

Many teenage girls as well as women of all ages have an unhealthy attitude where food is seen as the enemy. They are obsessed with looking perfect which is translated into being 'very thin'. The interesting thing is that this 'thinness' is not appealing to men but is lauded and praised by other women. For most of these women perfect bodies and food restriction is an obsession that could be called an 'disorder' of sorts but not quite in the category of serious mental illness.

Anorexia nervosa

This is an eating disorder in which a person severely restricts food intake and weighs at least 15 per cent less than her ideal weight. It usually is considered a female disorder, but anorexia nervosa occurs in men and is increasing in young boys. A person with this disorder fears being fat, and may be convinced that she is overweight despite what the scale shows or what other people say. To achieve skinniness, in addition to food restriction, she may use laxatives and exercise excessively. An anorexia sufferer is often very controlling and obsessive in other areas of her life, too. The problem usually begins in adolescence. In advanced stages of the illness, the dieting is hard to reverse. At that point, hunger may disappear completely and the pursuit of thinness becomes a way of life. Starvation causes medical complications of its own, such as thyroid problems, anaemia and joint pains. Death can occur in the most severe cases.

The causes are not clear. It is likely to be a combination of genetic and environmental factors. Some of the proposed causes include depression or anxiety or obsessive compulsive disorder, difficult family relationships, fears of adulthood and environmental pressures, such as images from glossy magazines, TV, etc.

Take charge, take care, take action
✦ A mental health professional, such as a psychiatrist, psychologist or social worker, must be seen as soon as you are concerned about yourself or a loved one. The earlier it is detected the better the prognosis.
✦ The health care professional will conduct a full history and assessment and will check the physical signs of starvation. Other tests may be done, including blood tests and kidney, liver and thyroid function.
✦ Some people have a single, relatively brief episode whereas for others, the problem becomes chronic and the person's condition gradually deteriorates. Anorexia is best treated with a combination of psychotherapy and medication Some people with anorexia nervosa may have to be hospitalised, either for treatment of medical complications or for treatment of the problematic behaviour related to food.

Bulimia nervosa
This is an eating disorder that involves binge eating: eating large quantities of food at one sitting, regardless of hunger. Most often, the condition also involves purging: the use of self-induced vomiting and/or abusing laxatives, suppositories, enemas or diuretics after a binge. Rather than purging, some people compensate for episodes of bingeing with other behaviours, such as fasting or overexercising. Bulimia mainly affects young women.

Although people with bulimia are afraid of becoming fat, most of them are of normal weight or slightly overweight. The foods on which they binge tend to be 'comfort foods' (sweet, pastries, ice cream etc). Like anorexia, bulimia can cause huge amounts of damage to your body. It can lead to dehydration from purging, chronic bowel problems from laxative use, tooth decay from excessive vomiting and gastrointestinal difficulties. It may even lead to permanent heart damage and death. Bulimia sufferers tend to feel very ashamed of themselves and they often show signs of addictive behaviour.

Many people with bulimia also have a history of anorexia or depression, anxiety and panic disorder. There is almost certainly a genetic predisposition to the disorder.

Take charge, take care, take action
+ As with anorexia, early detection is vital.
+ You must consult with a specialist, preferably a psychiatrist, who will do a full assessment and check you medically, too. Please be aware that bulimia can last for a short time or can continue for many years. Even after successful treatment, bulimia can return.
+ An eating disorder is a complex jumble of physical and emotional problems. Both must be addressed in order for treatment to work. Treatment must include psychological counselling, nutritional counselling and medication, such as antidepressants.
+ If someone you know shows signs of bulimia, contact a physician or mental health professional. Confronting someone with bulimia can be difficult. He or she may deny the problem or become defensive.

Binge-eating disorder
This is a recently classified disorder in which people have frequent episodes of compulsive overeating, but unlike those with bulimia, they do not purge their bodies of food. During these food binges, they often eat alone and very quickly, regardless of whether they feel hungry or full. They often feel shame or guilt over their actions. Unlike anorexia and bulimia, binge-eating disorder occurs almost as often in men as in women.

Endometriosis

This increasingly common condition is one of the major causes of infertility, and causes many women much distress and pain. The endometrium is the soft tissue that lines your uterus. Normally, this endometrial tissue alternately thickens and sheds each month with your period. But in some women, part of the endometrial tissue moves outside the uterus and starts to grow on and around other pelvic organs, such as the ovaries and Fallopian tubes or the colon and bladder.

Just like endometrial tissue inside the uterus, this external endometrial tissue thickens and bleeds monthly in response to release of estrogen. It causes painful cramps and heavy monthly bleeding. This endometrial tissue may exert pressure on the organs and result in pain, and the bleeding into the organs causes fibrosis and adhesions. Endometriosis may also lead to painful sexual intercourse, infertility or both.

The reason for the onset of endometriosis is not completely known. It is much more common in young successful professional women. The reason for this is unknown.

Take charge, take care, take action

✦ Empower yourself with as much information as possible. There are endometriosis centres at some private hospitals as well as Endo support groups which may be helpful.

✦ This condition is thought to be exacerbated by chemical residues called dioxins which are released into the environment as by-products of industrial processes. They are consumed by animals, then stored in fat tissues and therefore found in meat, fish and poultry, dairy products, and eggs. A diet with less animal fat and more green and leafy vegetables and complex carbohydrates is recommended. This will lead to a slightly lower level of these compounds in your body.

✦ If the endometrial tissue has encroached into your bowel area, make sure you avoid constipation and bloating, otherwise you may feel a lot worse. Be sure to eat plenty of vegetables and high-fibre foods, and drink lots of water to keep your bowels moving.

✦ A regular exercise programme can help relieve pain and cramps. Exercise reduces menstrual flow and thereby the endometrial irritation and inflammation. It also increases your body's production of endorphins. Walking is a good basic exercise though some women with endometriosis may find it more comfortable to swim or engage in stretching exercises and yoga.

✦ Painful sexual intercourse is a common complaint in endometriosis sufferers. Often just choosing a different position may help. The missionary position is not the best. The female on top is better as the woman has greater control over penetration. Experiment to find the most comfortable position.

✦ The pain of endometriosis can be severe, especially during menstruation. The best relief is usually achieved with a non-steroidal anti-inflammatory agent such as Ibuprofen.

✦ Chronic pain causes a release of stress hormones, which in turn increases pain sensitivity and it becomes a vicious cycle. Relaxation techniques such as chronic progressive muscle relaxation, guided imagery, breathing and meditation, may assist in breaking this cycle of pain and stress.

✦ The treatment for endometriosis ranges from hormone therapy to surgery. Together with your doctor, decisions can be made regarding the best treatment for you. Do not give up hope of conceiving. There is help at hand.

Glucose

Commonly referred to as blood sugar, a high blood glucose test (performed after a 10-hour fast) either indicates the presence or the possibility of developing diabetes. It is easy for your doctor to do a dipstick test of your urine and if it shows an abnormality to then do a fasting blood glucose test. It is a good idea to perform a blood glucose test every five years as a screening procedure. It is even more important to do this if you have a family history of diabetes. By the time diabetes is diagnosed, damage may have already occurred in various organs such as the eye, nervous system and kidneys. By the early testing and detection of a raised glucose, you may prevent the onset of diabetes or at least prevent damage to the organs in your body.

Headaches and migraines

Many more women than men are chronic headache sufferers. Chronic headaches mean you experience frequent headaches, for some sufferers almost every day!

Headaches can be classified into vascular and non-vascular headaches. 'Vascular' means the origin of the pain is from your blood vessels. Vascular headaches include migraines and cluster headaches. Non-vascular headaches are mostly caused by tension. This is the most common type of headache. Other non-vascular headaches may be due to dental, sinus or middle-ear infections. They are also commonly caused by a problem with the TMJ (tempero-mandibular joint).

The brain as a source of pain is extremely rare. The pain of a headache comes from outside the brain, because brain tissue does not have sensory nerves. The pain is from the scalp, the blood vessels and especially stretched and tensed muscles.

Tension headaches

These are not caused by disease, and are often considered to be 'normal' headaches. Tension headaches may be episodic or chronic (which occur more than 10 times per month). The pain is typically dull, steady, starts at the back of your head and spreads over your entire head. It is classically thought to be caused by a tightening of the muscles of face, neck and scalp, commonly due to poor posture, muscle tension and stress. The tightening of the muscles is thought to cause pinching of nerves and blood vessels, creating a sensation of pain and pressure. A scientific view proposes that these headaches are rather caused by changes in brain chemicals, which trigger pain from nerves and blood vessels.

Migraines

Two-thirds of people who get migraines are women, probably because of the influence of hormones. Migraines tend to run in families and frequently first appear during childhood or adolescence. A typical migraine headache is throbbing or pulsating, and is usually associated with an aura of nausea and visual disturbances, such as blurring and seeing stars, before the onset of the pain. Scientists still do not do not know exactly why migraines occur. The pain of migraines almost certainly results from swelling in blood vessels and nerves that surround the brain. This swelling is probably triggered by changes in brain chemicals and electrical activity. Women who have migraines often find that their headaches occur or worsen around the time of their menstrual periods. The two types of medications to treat migraines are those that are taken when a headache starts (abortive medications) and those that are taken every day to prevent migraines (preventive medications). The decision whether to take a daily preventive medication or abortive medications is a personal choice but one which you should discuss with your doctor.

Headache triggers
+ Certain foods, odours, menstrual periods and changes in weather are among many factors that may trigger your headache.
+ Stress as well as emotional factors such as depression, anxiety, frustration and even pleasant excitement may be associated with developing a headache.

Take charge, take care, take action
+ Keeping a headache diary will help you determine whether factors such as food, menstruation, change in weather, and/or mood have any relationship to your headache pattern. Lack of sleep or disrupted sleep patterns may also trigger migraines or tension headaches.
+ Cut back on alcohol and caffeine.
+ Diet may play a role in some individuals sensitive to a substance called tyramine which is found in red wine, cheese and some fish.
+ Some people are able to manage their tension headaches without medications.
+ Using a heating pad or a cold compress can be extremely helpful, or a massage to any tight areas in the neck and shoulders.

✦ Relaxation techniques, such as meditation and deep-breathing exercises or acupuncture, may help to decrease the frequency of headaches.

✦ For an occasional headache over-the-counter preparations such as aspirin, paracetomol or anti-inflammatories are very useful. But they may become habit-forming. Use of any over-the-counter pain reliever should be limited to no more than twice a week.

✦ Seventy per cent of chronic headaches are due to a phenomenon called 'rebound headaches' which are induced by the analgesics (painkillers). Heavy analgesic users experience headaches of much greater intensity and frequency.

✦ If you get severe chronic headaches, a daily preventive medication may help. Even for people without depression, a small dose of antidepressant medication has offered significant relief from chronic headache pain. (Discuss this with your doctor.)

Although very few headaches are signs of serious underlying medical conditions, call your doctor at once if any of the items below apply to you.

✦ You have three or more headaches per week.

✦ You must take a pain reliever every day or almost daily.

✦ You need more than recommended doses of over-the-counter medications to relieve headache symptoms.

✦ You have a stiff neck and/or fever in addition to a headache.

✦ Your headache is accompanied by shortness of breath, fever, and/or unexpected symptoms that affect your eyes, ears, nose or throat.

✦ You are dizzy, unsteady or have slurred speech, weakness or changes in sensation (numbness and/or tingling) in addition to your headache.

✦ You experience confusion or drowsiness with your headache.

✦ Your headaches begin and persist after a head injury.

✦ Your headache is triggered by exertion, coughing, bending or sexual activity.

✦ Your headache keeps getting worse and won't go away.

✦ Persistent or severe vomiting accompanies headache.

Heart disease

Heart disease is on the increase throughout the world, especially in developing countries. Although South Africa has always had a high incidence of ischaemic heart disease in certain population groups, the incidence has increased dramatically and it now affects everyone. (Ischaemic heart disease means blockages have occurred in coronary vessels which means less oxygen is getting to the heart.)

At the simplest level, the function of the heart is to pump blood. If the coronary arteries are in any way compromised, the heart muscle pump becomes inefficient, which in turn affects the whole body (see also page 280).

With a little knowledge about your heart and what is good or bad for it, you can significantly reduce your risk for heart disease.

As a woman your risk for a heart attack is minimal until you reach menopause when it becomes equal to that of a man. The hormone oestrogen has a cardio-protective effect. Around menopause the production of this hormone diminishes and your heart is no longer protected. You therefore need to take special care of your heart throughout your life, especially once you reach this stage. Women are more likely than men to die from a first heart attack and more likely to develop a second heart attack. The reason for this is that they are not as alert to the symptoms of heart disease and do not call for help as quickly as men. Do not ignore chest pain, shortness of breath and palpitations. Women experiencing angina or a heart attack often present with a slightly different type of chest pain. The pain in a male is typically a left-sided, heavy, pressing pain which may radiate into his jaw, shoulder, arm and back. Women, however, often experience this pain as a burning sensation and dismiss it as indigestion.

Heart disease and stroke are classified as chronic diseases of lifestyle. This means they arise as a result of bad lifestyle choices, such as an unhealthy diet, smoking and lack of exercise. Be watchful of your children's lifestyle factors, too.

Risk factors for coronary artery disease include the following:

✦ High blood pressure   ✦ High cholesterol

298

✦ Diabetes
✦ Cigarette smoking
✦ Physical inactivity.

✦ Family history
✦ Obesity

Take charge, take care, take action
Do all you can proactively to prevent heart disease, especially as you approach menopause and beyond. Manage all your risk factors for heart disease aggressively, particularly if you already have some signs of heart disease.
✦ Quit smoking
✦ Eat a healthy diet
✦ Reduce your high cholesterol
✦ Reduce high blood pressure
✦ Lose weight
✦ Exercise
✦ Prevent and treat diabetes.

There are two simple preventive medications that you can take if you are at high risk. First discuss with your doctor:
1. Ask about taking a daily mini-aspirin. This has a protective effect by thinning the blood and preventing clotting.
2. Ask your doctor about folic acid supplementation. This supplement may reduce some of the risk factors associated with heart disease. It has an effect on a substance called homocysteine.

If you have existing coronary artery disease you will need to be carefully monitored by your physician, with regular clinical check-ups, ECGs, stress ECGs and echocardiography. You will also be put onto appropriate medication according to your needs, including a combination of some of the following: cholesterol lowering meds, aspirin, calcium channel blockers, beta blockers, nitrates and antihypertensives.

HIV/AIDS
AIDS (Acquired Immune Deficiency Syndrome) was first described in the early 1980s. HIV (Human Immunodeficiency Virus) was discovered as the cause of AIDS in 1983. It is still unclear exactly where the virus originated.

Factors that have caused the virus to spread rapidly include socioeconomic instability, multiple sexual partner activity, as well as intravenous drug usage and migration of people across large distances. HIV is generally spread in three ways: via sexual intercourse, with HIV-infected blood directly into the body, and from mother to child transmission during pregnancy, childbirth and via breastfeeding. HIV is not spread by casual, everyday non-sexual contact. It is not spread by kissing, hugging or touching. Neither is it spread by handshaking, sharing food utensils or from toilet seats.

The HIV virus attacks and slowly destroys the immune system. There are three stages during the infection – being well with no symptoms, mild disease episodes and then very severe illness. Some people are rapid progressors (disease progresses and becomes very active) whereas others are slow progressors (they remain generally very well often for 10-15 years).

In South Africa the virus has spread rapidly leaving devastation in its wake. At least 4.5-million South Africans live with HIV. Close to a thousand HIV-related deaths occur per day, and there are currently at least 800 000 HIV orphans. There is an estimated HIV prevalence rate of 27.9% amongst sexually active women aged from 15-49, while the estimated general population HIV prevalence rate is 11.4%. With this exceptionally high HIV prevalence in South Africa, tremendous challenges exist in the fields of HIV education, prevention and care.

For women in particular this is a huge issue. Unfortunately, women often have very little control over their sexual lives and are victims of exploitation and gender-based violence (see page 324). On top of all this, it is the women who care for the sick and shoulder the huge burden.

Take charge, take care, take action
There are important things to understand about HIV and women:
1. Women are at much higher risk for getting the virus. HIV is transmitted from men to women much more easily than from women to men.
2. A woman's risk of infection is even higher with anal intercourse, or if you have a vaginal infection.

3. Obviously your risk increases even more if your partner has other sex partners, has had sex with infected people, or has sex with men.

4. It is your right as a woman **always** to **protect yourself** against HIV infection. Having your sex partner use a condom every time can lower the chance of HIV infection. Other forms of birth control, such as birth control pills or diaphragms, do **not** provide protection.

5. Gynaecological problems can be early signs of HIV infection. Ulcers in the vagina, persistent candida infections, and severe pelvic inflammatory disease (PID) can be signs of HIV. Hormone changes, contraceptive pills or antibiotics can also cause these vaginal problems. So do **not** panic but **do** see your doctor to make sure you know the cause.

6. Women get more and different HIV effects than men. Women are more likely to get skin rashes and liver problems, and to experience body shape changes, as well as problems from the human papilloma virus.

7. **Get tested** Many women don't find out they have HIV until they become ill or get tested during pregnancy. If women don't get tested for HIV, they seem to get sick and die faster than men. But if they get tested and treated, they can live a long, quality life.

8. **Get treatment** Fortunately, antiretroviral (ARV) treatment is now available through the state. Make sure you get adequate treatment. There are side effects but with time you develop a tolerance to many of them. And with treatment you can extend your lifespan and possibly prevent 'full blown AIDS'.

9. **Get support** Use every bit of support you can, whether it is from family members, your doctor or your community. Many women are full-time parents in addition to dealing with their health and employment. This can make it more difficult to take medications and schedule medical appointments. With proper support, however, women do very well on HIV treatment.

10. There should be no stigma attached to having HIV. People do not feel ashamed if they have chronic diseases like diabetes, arthritis or cancer. So, too, if you are HIV-positive you

should not have to feel ashamed and should have access to good medical care. In some communities many women and girls who disclose their HIV status to partners, family members and communities are in danger of being physically and emotionally abused.

Although prevention of HIV is paramount, countless numbers of people in our country are already infected with the virus. With early diagnosis HIV has been transformed from a terrible death sentence to a chronic and manageable disease, and the quality of life can continue for many years.

Even if you are married and monogamous, every sexually active individual should go for an HIV test. Voluntary counselling and testing (VCT) is the best way to encourage early diagnosis and thereby improve care with positive wellness programmes that include an understanding of the disease, encouraging a healthy lifestyle, offering nutritional supplements, preventing and treating infections and access to appropriate, affordable and sustainable ARV therapy.

Hypertension (see Blood pressure)

Infertility

As a young woman you assume that when you want to have a child, you will simply fall pregnant. The average time taken for a couple trying to conceive is between 6-12 months of having frequent intercourse (see 'Trying to conceive' on page 315). Ten to fifteen per cent of couples will continue to have difficulty conceiving after one year of trying. When this happens, the couple is considered to have a problem with infertility. It is a 'couple' problem, not one or the other. The cause of infertility occurs about as often in men as in women and in about 20 per cent, both partners have a problem. In some infertile couples, no cause can be found to explain the problem.

Causes of infertility
Ovulatory causes
Ovulatory problems are the cause of infertility in about 20 per cent of cases. Common causes of ovulatory disorders include eating disorders,

unusually heavy exercise, rapid weight loss, low body weight and obesity, as well as hormonal abnormalities such as thyroid problems, pituitary gland problems, adrenal gland problems and Polycystic Ovary Syndrome (PCO). The natural process of ageing is also a factor to consider. It significantly affects the ease with which you become pregnant. Your ovaries and eggs become older as you age so that ovulation becomes slower and less effective.

Tubal causes
Fallopian tube damage is the cause of infertility in approximately 30 per cent of female problems. The damage may be due to tubal scarring from pelvic inflammatory disease (from sexually transmitted illnesses) or scarring from endometriosis. Damage to the tubes could be due to a previous ectopic pregnancy or previous surgery.

Abnormalities of the uterus
These account for almost 20 per cent of female infertility problems. Scar tissue within the lining of the uterus may arise from uterine infections, spontaneous or therapeutic abortions or surgical procedures such as a D&C.

Male infertility problems
These are manifest in abnormal sperm which means either a low sperm count or abnormal morphology (structure) or motility (movement) of the sperm. The causes include hormonal, testicular or sperm-flow problems, medications, drugs and anabolic steroids, toxic exposure, abnormal sperm function, chromosomal disorders or general illnesses. In up to 50 per cent of infertile men, no specific cause can be identified.

Take charge, take care, take action
✦ After one year of trying to conceive, it is a wise decision to get yourself and your partner checked out. You need to be referred to a specialist gynaecologist or specialised centre for infertility treatment. Unfortunately, most medical aids do not cover the often expensive treatments.

303

+ If you are over 35, you may want to consult your doctor after four to six months of trying to conceive and over 40 you should seek medical help sooner. Your doctor will review your medical history and conduct a thorough physical examination.
+ The investigations that will be done include ovulatory assessments (through checking your cervical mucous and your hormones at different times during your cycles) and a hysterosalpingogram (HSG) (x-ray study of uterus and tubes) and ultrasound scans.
+ The treatment depends on your specific problem. Surgery may be required to remove a fibroid tumour or medicines to treat an ovulation or hormonal problem. Ovulatory disorders can be treated with various hormonal or fertility medications. Artificial insemination (AI) or in vitro fertilisation (IVF) may need to be discussed as options.

It is an emotionally traumatic time for a couple. It is a long process involving a lot of medical tests and interventions that can go on for months and even many years. But because of dramatic improvements in technology and medication, it is possible for up to half of couples who seek infertility treatments to conceive. Even when there is no medical explanation for a couple's infertility, it's still possible that the couple may conceive.

It is always important to strengthen your body, your mind and your emotions. Make sure you eat a nutritious diet, that you exercise moderately and that you implement a stress-busting technique such as meditation as you go through this challenging time.

Irritable bowel syndrome

Irritable bowel syndrome, or IBS, is a condition characterised by abdominal cramping, bloating, gas, and other changes in the bowel habit, such as alternating periods of constipation or diarrhoea.

It is much more common in women. It is not clear what causes IBS. Excessive stress, changes in diet, emotional upsets or hormonal changes seem to be some of the factors that increase the symptoms associated with IBS. Medication may be required, such as antispasmodics to relieve bowel spasms, and medication to decrease nerve sensitivity in the bowels.

The long-term effects are often associated with frustration over the symptoms, and there does not seem to be any long-term damage to the stomach or intestines.

Take charge, take care, take action
It may be difficult to prevent but the following steps may help:
✦ Watch calorie intake
✦ Eat a diet low in fat
✦ Avoid gas producing foods such as cabbage, onions, mushrooms, cauliflower, spinach
✦ Cut down on caffeine, alcohol and artificial sweeteners
✦ Monitor fibre intake
✦ Manage stress and learn stress management techniques.

Libido
A fading libido is a common issue for women, especially those in long-term relationships. Sometimes the thrill is gone because your sex drive cannot peacefully coexist with stress, exhaustion, anger or marital discord. Women are indeed complicated and there is not going to be a magic bullet (like Viagra) that cures all women of sexual dysfunction. A purely physical approach will never work for a woman's libido, the reason being that emotions play a huge role and a woman's primary erogenous zone is the brain!

Take charge, take care, take action
Too tired
No matter what causes the fatigue – insomnia, working late or a new baby – the reality is that all you want to do when you fall into your bed *is sleep!*
✦ You can no longer rely on spontaneous sex. Make a date for sex. Speak about it in the morning so you both can think about sex and each other all day.
✦ Go to the gym together for 30-40 minutes one evening. Exercise is great to enhance and encourage sex. Your blood is circulating, your

nervous system is firing, so it makes for good sex (you will sleep well, too, following so much exertion!).

✦ Give each other time to catch a nap or to sleep in, and schedule some time during the weekend for connecting.

Relationship problems

Problems in the relationship manifest first in the bedroom. It is much easier to say *'I have a headache'* when the truth is *'I'm angry with you'*.

✦ Consider a few sessions of marital therapy, but don't try to deal with relationship issues by shutting down sexually. If you do, you'll both end up suffering.

✦ Women often use sex as a way of communicating their discontent or anger. Use vocabulary as opposed to withholding sex. Let your partner know that you want to talk about something important, and talk instead of withholding.

✦ Pay special attention to what your partner is saying, too.

After the baby

Over 80 per cent of women have some sexual dysfunction in the first year after they have given birth. Fatigue and the huge focus on your new baby do play a role in sidetracking your sex life, but most of it is hormonal. Breastfeeding definitely affects your libido and your ability to be aroused, and it can even make sex painful. Breastfeeding lowers your body's production of the hormones oestrogen and testosterone and the brain chemical dopamine. You can lose your desire for sex and your vaginal walls thin out and don't produce the lubrication you need for intercourse, so sex can hurt. (A similar problem occurs during menopause.) Also, the progesterone-only pill (mini-pill) that most women use as contraception during lactation makes things even worse.

✦ Use lots of lubrication. Many effective over-the-counter products are available and they really help. You can also speak to your doctor about using a small dose of vaginal oestrogen cream to thicken and moisten your vaginal lining.

✦ Catch up on rest. Sleep deprivation is a real libido dampener.

Hormonal life changes

Taking the oral contraceptive pill and especially going through menopause can dramatically disrupt your sex life. Many birth control pills lower testosterone and thereby lower libido. Although testosterone is the essential male hormone, it is produced in small amounts in healthy women and is essential for a strong libido. There is also a natural decline in testosterone from late 20s and it is significantly down by your 40s.

✦ Change to another contraceptive. Check out which pills don't dampen libido or consider another form of contraception, such as an intrauterine device which doesn't interfere with libido.

✦ Consider testosterone. Patches and creams are being used successfully especially in menopausal women or those following removal of ovaries. Many of the products are new and you must be guided by your gynaecologist. It may improve orgasm and arousal.

No orgasms/few orgasms

Do not believe everything you read. The vast majority of women do not and cannot achieve an orgasm with sexual intercourse. There must be some clitoral stimulation and it often takes time, patience and letting go. Don't forget that the group of antidepressants called SSRIs including Prozac, Arropax and Cipramil all decrease libido and inhibit orgasm.

✦ Slow it down: It can take a long time; slow down the whole sexual experience. Try other forms of clitoral stimulation.

✦ Initiate sex talk.

✦ Do something different!

Pain

Any kind of pain in your body can interfere with your sex life and diminish your libido. But the most common cause of pain in the genital region is due to lack of lubrication, which can make intercourse unbearable. It is mainly due to oestrogen decline during menopause and breastfeeding, as well as following surgical removal of the ovaries.

✦ Gynaecological conditions such as endometriosis, ovarian cancer or interstitial cystitis (inflammation of the bladder) can also cause pain during sex and especially at other times. Vulvodynia is a specific condition characterised by chronic pain and inflammation at the opening of the vagina. Some women may also have painful muscle spasms, often precipitated by childbirth, scoliosis or lower-back problems that lead to a lot of pain on intercourse. For all these serious conditions, see your gynaecologist or a specialist.

✦ Avoid irritants such as perfumed soaps, bubble baths and feminine hygiene sprays which can irritate the vagina.

Menopause

Menopause is not the beginning of the end! It is a time of renewal, a new cycle of your life. It is a natural event that normally occurs between the ages of 48 and 55, a transition from your childbearing years to a new stage of life in which your own personal needs and desires can take on a more central focus. While it may be a period of disequilibrium and emotional or physical discomfort, it may also facilitate a new state of equilibrium, a period of renewed energy and often a new sense of purpose. You, however, need to make a conscious positive choice to create this reality.

The essential issue in menopause is a deficiency of oestrogen. At this stage your ovarian function declines and oestrogen production diminishes. The symptoms do not suddenly begin at age 50 or with your last menstrual period. They can begin anywhere from two to 10 years before the cessation of periods. You may experience any combination of these symptoms:

✦ Hot flushes
✦ Night sweats
✦ Insomnia
✦ Mood swings including irritability, depression, and anxiety
✦ Irregular menstrual periods
✦ Spotting of blood in between periods
✦ Vaginal dryness and painful sexual intercourse
✦ Decreased sex drive
✦ Vaginal infections
✦ Urinary tract infections

✦ Blood and urine tests can be used to measure your hormone levels that may indicate whether you are close to menopause or within it.

In addition to these symptoms which can last anywhere from two to eight years, the long-term effects of menopause include bone loss and possible osteoporosis, as well as changes in cholesterol levels and greater risk of heart disease.

Take charge, take care, take action
Whether you choose hormone replacement therapy (HRT), herbal, homeopathic treatment, or no treatment at all, perhaps the more important issues are what health-enhancing choices and changes you can make through this transition.

✦ Empower yourself with knowledge and information. It is the 'not knowing' that holds women in the grip of fear. With knowledge comes the power to implement the strategies required to enhance your wellbeing.

✦ Regular exercise increases circulating oestrogen and significantly reduces hot flushes. It increases your energy levels, deepens REM sleep, blunts anxiety and depression and elevates your mood. It decreases your risk of heart disease and increases bone density, preventing osteoporosis.

✦ Reduce your intake of caffeine, alcohol, refined sugar and salt. Large meals as well as highly spicy foods dilate the blood vessels and exacerbate your hot flushes. Try to eat smaller meals more frequently.

✦ Frequent sex is good for both the relationship and for your health during menopause. Women experiencing intercourse at least once a week have twice as much circulating natural oestrogen than their non-sexually active counterparts. These women have a healthier vaginal mucosa, far fewer hot flushes and a better libido.

HRT or not?

Discuss with your doctor whether or not to take hormones to relieve your symptoms, weighing your risks against any possible benefits. Pay careful attention to the many options currently available to you that do not involve taking hormones. If you have a uterus and decide to take estrogen, you must also take progesterone to prevent endometrial cancer (cancer of the lining of the uterus). If you do not have a uterus, progesterone is not necessary.

HRT is excellent for treating and eliminating menopausal symptoms, and also protects your bones from osteporosis and has always been thought to provide a cardioprotective effect. But very recent studies have confirmed the slightly increased risk of possible breast cancer and possibly not very much cardiac protection, perhaps even a detrimental affect. (There will be many forthcoming studies needed to confirm these findings.) It is, however, still highly effective in preventing osteoporosis and possibly other cancers.

Nothing is as effective as oestrogen replacement for oestrogen deficiency symptoms. HRT is advocated for short-term use (two to five years) rather than previously recommended for many years postmenopausally. It is also recommended that you use the lowest possible dosage required and must have close monitoring with frequent and regular physical exams, including breast exams and mammograms.

Herbal or botanical preparations have been shown to ease some of the symptoms and are even being advocated by gynaecologists. There are many products available in South Africa containing substances such as licorice root, black cohosh, gingko biloba and angelica sinensis. Please discuss the option of taking herbal or homeopathic medication with your doctor. Even herbal preparations have side effects and possible toxicity, so be aware of what you take.

Migraine (see Headaches)

Obesity

Obesity is characterised by excessive fat storage and it's one of the most common health problems in both developed and developing countries. It has become a global crisis, escalating in children as well as in adults. It often increases your risk of diseases such as diabetes, hypertension (high blood pressure), arthritis and cancer. It is well known that obesity is associated with feeling depressed, anxious and miserable. Obesity is diagnosed by calculating your body mass index (BMI). BMI is calculated using your height and weight. A BMI of 30 or more defines obesity (see Chapter 4, page 189).

Take charge, take care, take action
+ Crash diets do not work. A combination of dietary therapy, physical activity and behavioural therapy is necessary.
+ You certainly need direction, guidance and the support of a nutrition therapist and/or your doctor.
+ Moderate levels of physical activity 30-45 minutes a day, three to five days a week is recommended. The activity should be started slowly and gradually increased in intensity.

Follow the tips with regard to nutrition (Chapter 3) and exercise (Chapter 4) and make sure you are staying mentally fit at the same time. A slow weight loss by reducing fat intake and refined starch and sugars, combined with a simple exercise such as brisk walking, will improve your general body condition, your mood and your mental state.

Osteoporosis
Osteoporosis is a common condition in South African women. It is a progressive disease in which the bones gradually become weaker, and is associated with loss of bone density and thinning bone tissue. It is a silent and painless disease, primarily affecting women after menopause when the hormone oestrogen begins to decline. The lack of oestrogen triggers an increase in bone resorption, i.e. bone loss. The average woman begins to lose bone mass from about age 35; those who have been physically active are far less prone to osteoporosis.

The risk factors for osteoporosis include a thin body frame, women who smoke and drink alcohol, and lack of exercise. While osteoporosis causes no specific symptoms until it is advanced, some early warning signs include a gradual loss of height and a stooping of shoulders. Eventually the bones will fracture, causing significant problems in many areas from the spine to the wrists.

Take charge, take care, take action
+ Did you know that osteoporosis is almost entirely preventable? But don't only start thinking about it at 45! The earlier you think about it, the better. Eat calcium-rich foods and engage in regular weight-bearing exercise.
+ For good self-care, especially while you are younger, make sure you are taking sufficient calcium, exercising regularly and eating a well-balanced diet. It is best to take calcium in a formulation, together with magnesium in a dosage of at least 800 micrograms of calcium daily. and eat good quality low-fat dairy products. Cut back on coffee and alcohol. They both leech calcium from your bones.

Pain

Everyone experiences pain throughout their lives for different reasons. You have pain receptors in every part of your body. You accidentally touch a hot stove and in a split second, you pull your hand away. How? The pain receptors send electrical messages through your spinal cord to the brain. In this case the pain is useful. It sends a message of danger. It begins suddenly and doesn't last long.

Chronic pain, however, is persistent and disturbs your daily function. It is usually due to injury and inflammation to any part of the body. It usually lasts a month or more, and could last years. Chronic pain can come and go many times or remain constant and it can disturb sleep patterns, decrease appetite and cause depression.

The most common chronic pain is that of the musculoskeletal system, especially back or neck pain, joint pain or arthritis. Other causes are severe headaches or migraines and gut and stomach pains.

People 50 and older are twice as likely as those under 50 to have been diagnosed with chronic pain. Women are more likely than men to be chronic pain sufferers.

Take charge, take care, take action
+ Different people tolerate different degrees of pain but you should never ignore pain. Consult a doctor if you cannot determine why you

are experiencing pain, especially if it continues relentlessly or if it doesn't respond to simple treatment.

✦ Once the cause of pain is diagnosed, it may be possible to prevent it from coming back. For example, people diagnosed with gastrointestinal disorders can change their diets to help prevent pain.

✦ Taking medication is still the most commonly used method of relief from pain. Over-the-counter medications, such as paracetomol, are the most commonly used analgesics (painkillers). Aspirin and anti-inflammatories such as ibuprofen (brufen) work by interfering with pain messages, and by reducing inflammation, swelling and irritation that can make pain worse.

✦ Sometimes prescription medication such as stronger anti-inflammatories or higher schedule painkillers, may be prescribed by your doctor. Other meds such as anaesthetics, antidepressants and corticosteroids, may work against certain types of pain. Sometimes medications are injected directly into the region of pain or near a nerve to interrupt the pain signal. Narcotic pain relievers, such as codeine, are among the most powerful pain treatments and are only used for short periods for severe, intense pain as they are highly addictive. Morphine is reserved for the most intense pain associated with cancer.

✦ It is important that you only use what is recommended by your doctor and are aware that many painkillers are habit-forming and have significant side effects.

Taking excessive amounts of painkillers can often make pain worse, for example, rebound headaches.

Non-drug treatments for pain
More and more people are using non-drug modalities to treat pain, many of which are highly effective. If you suffer from chronic pain, try one of these different therapies:

✦ Acupuncture
✦ Exercise and physiotherapy
✦ Massage
✦ Relaxation and meditation
✦ Psychotherapy
✦ Herbal remedies.

In some cases, these treatments may stimulate natural painkillers, called endorphins, which are created within the body. In other cases, non-drug treatments work directly on nerves to interfere with pain messages.

Pap smear (cervical health)

Cancer of the cervix is a totally preventable disease.With the use of Pap smear results, any abnormal cells can be treated right away and cancer prevented.

This simple screening measure should be done every year from the time that you are sexually active until your later years.

Take charge, take care, take action

✦ Go to your family doctor, gynaecologist or local clinic for this simple investigation which can save your life.
✦ The latest breakthrough news is the discovery of a vaccine against HPV (human papilloma virus) which is the cause of cervical cancer. This is a remarkable milestone but it will take quite a while until it is routinely offered to all women. Up until that time you must continue to go for yearly Pap smears.

Pregnancy care

From conception to the delivery of a healthy baby, there is a great deal that you can do to ensure optimal health. Most women do not even think about achieving best health until after falling pregnant, but it is important to begin to take extra care as soon as you decide to start trying to conceive. Good pre- and periconception care can significantly improve the quality of the pregnancy and ensure a happy outcome for both the infant and mother.

Take charge, take care, take action
Preconception
Make sure to optimise your nutrition and stay physically fit. If you are extremely overweight, consider trying to shed some extra kilos before

conception. It is wise to have a chat and a check-up with your doctor to ensure that your blood pressure, urine and general health is good. It is highly recommended that you take folic acid supplementation (400 micrograms daily). This has been shown to have a protective effect on the very early brain and neural tube development in the foetus. You are also advised to avoid all medications, unless they are necessary and recommended by your doctor, and to avoid all alcohol and drug use. Research shows that occasional alcohol consumption is not problematic but keep it to the occasional glass of wine. Stop smoking. Even herbal preparations and common over-the-counter medications may interfere with normal development of the foetus so first check everything with your doctor.

Trying to conceive

It takes a healthy fertile couple an average of six and often up to twelve months of trying, before conception takes place. Obviously there are lucky couples who conceive in the first month or two. But do not get distressed if nothing has happened immediately. If nothing happens after 6-12 months, consult your doctor. Even then it does not necessarily mean there is an infertility problem. (See Infertility, page 302.) You may just need some reassurance.

Monitor your fertile days

If you are willing to take some extra steps, you can monitor two body functions to pinpoint your most fertile times, maximising your chances of getting pregnant. The changes in the consistency of your cervical fluid and your body temperature are the two indicators of fertility.

1. **The cervical fluid** comprises the normal physiological discharge from your vagina. You will notice through your cycle that it changes in colour, amount and consistency. It will be slippery and stretchy on your most fertile days. At the beginning of your cycle, there is almost no discharge at all. Then it may become sticky or gummy, and then creamy and white. Finally, as ovulation approaches, it becomes more clear and stretchy, almost like egg white. Your cervical fluid actually gives you advance notice that you are about to ovulate. Another sign

on fertile days is the wet sensation felt inside the lower end of the vagina.

2. **Body temperature.** This is not completely accurate but does provide a guideline.

Use a thermometer to take your temperature. Create a chart and write down your temperature every day. From one day to the next, your temperature will fluctuate a little. These small temperature changes will seem random at first – ignore them. Take your temperature at the same time every morning before you get out of bed and keep the thermometer in your mouth for five minutes. After you ovulate, your body temperature will rise and stay at an elevated level for the rest of your ovulation cycle. At the end of your cycle, it falls again.

Ovulation predictor kit. This tests a hormone in your urine called Luteining Hormone (LH) and is very accurate. You can buy these kits from many pharmacies.

Just pregnant

Once you suspect that you may be pregnant because you have missed your period, testing can be done by your doctor with a urine or blood test or you can use a home pregnancy test kit available from most pharmacies. But please note that this should be done after your first missed period and even then you may occasionally still find that the test is negative. This will need to be followed up a few days later. Other early signs of pregnancy include breast tenderness, darkening of your nipples and areolae, and the formation of little bumps around your nipples that are called Montgomery's tubercles. You will also probably feel nauseous and fatigued.

Once you have confirmed your pregnancy, you will be seen by your doctor or clinic sister regularly to ensure the best prenatal care. This includes:

✦ Frequent prenatal examinations to detect early problems. Prenatal visits are typically scheduled:

☆ every four weeks during the first 32 weeks

★ every two weeks from 32 to 36 weeks

★ weekly from 36 weeks to delivery.

✦ Weight gain, blood pressure, height of your uterus and the foetal heartbeat are usually measured and recorded at each visit, and routine urine screening tests are performed.

✦ Other investigations include:

★ ultrasound scans to detect the foetal heart and the possibility of any problems

★ routine screening for:

☆ urine infections

☆ blood group testing

☆ rubella (german measles) immunity

☆ sexually transmitted diseases

☆ genetic screening (if there is a family history or if you are older than 35 years)

☆ blood pressure abnormalities

☆ protein in urine.

✦ Throughout the three trimesters of your pregnancy, make sure to take excellent care of yourself. Eat a nourishing diet by following the SELF **diet** outlined in chapter 3. You do not need to eat for two!

✦ If you are exercising regularly at the time of conception, you may carry on with your regular schedule until near the end. But do not do anything that raises your body temperature excessively.

✦ If you are unfit, consider beginning gentle exercise classes. There are many designed specially for pregnant women. Or begin swimming or walking regularly.

✦ Try and fit in some extra rest, even if it is just elevating your legs at the end of a busy work day and doing some gentle breathing exercises.

✦ Continue to enjoy a satisfying sex life through your pregnancy. It is in no way harmful to your foetus. In fact, many women have a surge in libido while pregnant. The only time you need to be cautious is if you have had a threatened miscarriage or have sutures (stitches) in your cervix. Then be advised by your doctor.

Premenstrual syndrome (PMS)

Menstruation involves the lining of the uterus (under hormonal control by the hypothalamus, pituitary gland and ovaries) and lasts roughly 28 days. This time period can vary greatly between individuals. Some women can have short cycles of 26 days or less whereas others go on for up to 35 days and beyond. Many women also have unpredictable and irregular cycles which is really not serious most of the time. If the egg is not fertilised (as in the majority of cycles), it dies, the uterus sheds its lining, bleeding begins and another menstrual cycle ensues.

PMS describes a group of symptoms and signs that occur in relation to the menstrual cycle and which interfere with a woman's life. The symptoms usually begin five to 11 days before the start of menstruation. Symptoms should stop when menstruation begins, or shortly thereafter. PMS is estimated to affect up to 75 per cent of women during their childbearing years.

The exact cause of PMS has not been identified, but we do know that it is related to hormonal shifts during your cycle. It seems to get worse as you age and approach menopause. Unfortunately, bad PMS sufferers seem to have a more difficult menopause and have a greater risk of postnatal depression. The most common physical and emotional symptoms include:

✦ abdominal cramps and bloating
✦ headaches
✦ swelling of feet, ankles and hands
✦ breast tenderness
✦ backaches
✦ weight gain
✦ cold sores or mouth ulcers
✦ constipation or diarrhoea
✦ food cravings (especially carbohydrates)
✦ anxiety or panic
✦ depression
✦ irritability
✦ weepiness

✦ hostility or aggression
✦ loss of libido
✦ sluggishness, lethargy.

Take charge, take care, take action
✦ Do not just dismiss any symptom that you may be experiencing
(especially the emotional symptoms) as PMS. Make sure that if these
symptoms last for longer than a few days and are not relieved with
onset or after menstruation that your doctor looks out for other
causes of the symptoms.
✦ Regular exercise is essential throughout your cycle. It eases both the
physical and the emotional symptoms.
✦ In addition to a really healthy diet (increased wholegrains,
vegetables, fruit, and decreased salt, sugar, alcohol and caffeine), add
supplements to help you.Vitamin B6, calcium, magnesium, zinc,
vitamin E and omega-3 oils have been shown to assist with relieving
symptoms.
✦ With excessive pain, aspirin and meds such as ibuprofen are very
effective. In severe fluid retention your doctor may prescribe a
diuretic for a day or two. Some women experience such severe
emotional disturbances that a condition called PMDD (premenstrual
dysphoric disorder) has been classified. These women may need
psychiatric medications or psychotherapy.
✦ Herbal and botanical therapies have been shown to assist with
symptoms. Angelica sinensis, predominantly regarded as a 'female'
remedy, is thought to be effective in both PMS and menopause, as
well as glycyrrhiza glabra (liquorice root) useful for water retention
and black cohosh for mood swings and irritability. Check these out
with your doctor first and avoid liquorice root if you have hypertension.

Smoking
Smoking is such a difficult habit to break, but by cutting down or even
better, stopping completely, you have the power to change your future
dramatically. It is the single most important risk factor.

You are aware that smoking is damaging, but do you know just how destructive it is to your health? Smoking changes the composition of your blood and therefore affects your circulation. Your chance of having a heart attack is more than double, and you have a fourteen times risk of developing lung cancer than non-smokers. You are also at very high risk of developing a whole host of other diseases including strokes, vascular disease and gangrene, as well as some awful cancers of the mouth, throat, nose and bladder.

The good news is that by making the decision to stop, you can dramatically reduce your risk of developing these awful conditions and you can save what is left of your good lung function and allow some areas to return to normal.

Tobacco kills about three million people a year and greatly outstrips all other causes of premature death.

It is never too late to quit because in one year after quitting, the risk of heart disease is halved and within approximately 10 years, the risk is as if you had never smoked.

Take charge, take care, take action
The most successful way to quit smoking is to make a plan and follow through with it.
+ Clear your house of cigarettes, lighters and ashtrays. Clean your house in order to eliminate any lingering odors.
+ Avoid the places that you associate with smoking, for example, your particular spot outside your office or a specific coffee shop. Also try to avoid standing next to or being with smokers.
+ During moments of intense craving, do something to distract yourself.
+ Try to do this together with someone else. Someone who is also trying to quit can help you try stick to your goal.
+ Tell your friends and family what you're doing and ask them all to help you through it.

Sexuality (see Libido)

Stress in women

Stress is a normal part of life. And I would suggest even more so for women who carry more of the load at home, within the extended family and the community together with the demands in the workplace. A certain amount of stress is necessary and even good for you. This 'good stress' is better called 'challenge'. You need the challenge of work, goals and vision to keep you motivated and focused.

Unfortunately, every-day stress often becomes overwhelming. It is when the stressful situation becomes unrelenting that damage begins to occur. As your worries envelop you, there is an outpouring of stress hormones which wear out the adrenal gland and deplete the immune system. This may cause you to develop health problems: the vast majority of illnesses are either directly caused or triggered by stress. It is important to recognise the signs of overwhelming stress and to deal with it.

The specific body (physiological) changes that occur in stressful situations are called the 'fight-flight' reaction. The primitive response of your body to stress is either to flee or to fight (see page 210). As soon as your body experiences a danger or perceived danger (stress) it starts to mobilise its forces. Your body responds in an identical manner whether you are actually in danger or just thinking about it. The problem is that this response goes on relentlessly within your body even when there is no danger, just deadlines, bills to pay, work to be completed and chores to be attended to all at a frenetic pace. The adrenalin continues to pump and the stress simmers away inside you.

It is normal to feel anxious, stressed and even depressed some of the time. If these feelings seem to be present with you most of the time, it is important to seek help from a psychologist.

Take care, take charge, take action

In the midst of all this external chaos, you have the power to create internal harmony instead of internal tension. The value of learning potent stress management techniques provides your body with the physiological experience to fight off stress. It allows your mind and body time to repair, regenerate and recover from the wear and tear of every-day strain.

✦ Rest and adequate quality sleep are essential to withstand and manage stress. Sleep is a time for restoring and repairing all the wear and tear effect of stress, both emotionally and physically.
✦ Use some easy breathing techniques often throughout the day to calm your nervous system.
✦ Learn a relaxation technique, such as meditation or visualisation, to implement into your daily strategy. It provides your body with the experience opposite to stress i.e. calm, tranquillity and peace for a short period every day.
✦ Exercise is a great stress buster. It blows off excessive agitation and negative energy.
✦ Communicate: Being able to offload to someone who can truly listen to you is extremely beneficial.

Urinary tract infection (see Bladder problems)

Vaginal discharges/infections
Vaginal discharge is a fluid coming from the vagina, normally clear, cloudy or whitish. The consistency and amount of discharge varies during your menstrual cycle. The vagina normally contains bacteria as well as fungal organisms, and a healthy vagina keeps a balance of these bacteria and fungi. Bacterial growth is controlled and affected by many different factors, such as acid level (pH) and hormones. Anything that upsets this balance may increase your risk of infection or overgrowth of any of the normal bacteria or by yeast. Possible triggers include:
✦ Antibiotic use
✦ Birth-control pills
✦ Douching
✦ Diabetes
✦ Pregnancy
✦ Stress
✦ Tight or synthetic undergarments
What indicates an *abnormal discharge or vaginitis* (inflammation of the vagina)?

+ itching
+ burning
+ offensive-smelling discharge
+ a yellowish or greenish colour
+ painful vagina, especially during intercourse
+ discomfort and burning during intercourse
+ swelling or redness of the lips of the vagina
+ discomfort or burning with urination.

Causes of an abnormal discharge

+ **Candida,** or thrush (a yeast infection), is the most common. Most women experience at least one bout of candida in their lifetime.
+ **Bacterial vaginosis,** commonly caused by a change in the normal bacteria of the vagina. This does not mean it is a sexually transmitted infection. It includes Gardnerella, a type of bacteria found normally in the female genital tract and Trichomonas, a type of parasite.
+ **Atrophic vaginitis** – irritation of the vagina that causes burning and dryness (common at menopause).
+ **A foreign body** in the vagina, such as a forgotten tampon or infection with the intrauterine device (IUD).
+ **Sexually transmitted Infections** (STIs), such as gonorrhea, genital herpes, or chlamydia.

Take charge, take care, take action
It is important that you do not ignore a vaginal discharge. It probably will not go away on its own and a sexually transmitted infection can develop into *pelvic inflammatory disease* which involves the structures within your pelvis, especially your Fallopian tubes, which is serious. You do need to see your doctor for an abnormal discharge. He or she will need to perform a pelvic examination using a device called a speculum to look at the cervix directly. During the pelvic exam, a sample of discharge is collected for testing in a laboratory.

A vaginal discharge from a bacterial or yeast infection responds to treatment with antibiotics or antifungals (depending on infection) within a few days to a week. Sexually transmitted diseases also should respond to antibiotic treatment within a week. If the infection progresses to pelvic inflammatory disease beyond the vaginal area, it may take much longer to treat.

With sexually transmitted infections, your partner will need to be treated too. Be aware that with multiple partners, you run a high risk of developing many sexually transmitted infections and HIV. Use condoms, practise safe sex and seriously consider changing your lifestyle.

Violence against women (gender-based violence)

Gender-based violence, or violence against women, is a major public health and human rights problem throughout the world. On average, a woman is raped in South Africa every minute. It is estimated that about one in every three women will be a victim of rape in their lifetime. This translates to more than 1000 women being raped daily. Such violence is pervasive in all societies and in South Africa is a particularly serious problem. The World Health Organisation classifies VAW (Violence Against Women) into two categories.

1. Violence against women by an intimate male partner or ex-partner, which is known as domestic violence. This category includes physical and sexual violence, emotional abuse, and a range of coercive behaviours. In South Africa, one adult woman out of every six is assaulted regularly by her mate.
2. The second category is sexual violence, which includes rape and other forms of sexual coercion, either by partners or by others.

Violence against women also interacts with the HIV epidemic in many ways. Obviously it is always unprotected intercourse and often more physical trauma to the vagina is possible than with consensual sex. Many committed rapes are performed by gangs, thereby increasing the viral exposure, and the prevalence of the HIV virus in rapists is high.

Take charge, take care, take action
+ Gender-based violence is everyone's issue.
+ Know that you are not powerless and you are not alone. If you are in

an abusive relationship, it is not your fault so do not feel shame. You are not trapped and there IS a way to get out. There are many organisations to help you, such as POWA (People Opposing Woman Abuse).

+ Being cautious, such as not driving alone at night, not talking to strangers or not accepting a lift, may cause you to be less vulnerable. But it does not mean that you should live in fear, or that altering your lifestyle will make you safe from attack. It does mean that you should be aware of the problem and make minor changes when possible. Learn to assess your particular situation and plan ahead.

+ The matter of rape should never be passed over lightly. It essential to try and report the incident. There are many really caring and efficient rape clinics where the reporting, examination and testing is all done in a very sensitive manner. You can ask to have a female doctor, nurse or other woman present during the examination. The doctor may offer a tranquilliser and will test for sexually transmitted infections and HIV. HIV prophylaxis must also be given. It is essential to receive psychological counselling after this traumatic experience.

Bibliography

In addition to many years of medical study and clinical experience, several books have impacted on my perception and understanding of health, life and medicine over the years. Some of the concepts have been mentioned within SELF.

I present them here as a means for you to broaden your outlook and enhance your life.

Chopra, Deepak: *Ageless Body, Timeless Mind*. Harmony Books, 1993
Evian, Clive: *Primary Aids Care 3rd edition*. Johannesburg: Jacana
    Education, 2000
Gafni, Marc: *Soul Print*. Penguin Books, 2001
Ganong, W.F: *Review of Medical Physiology*. Appleton and Lange, 2000
Greenberg, A. *The Wings of the Sun*. Breslov Research Institute, 1995
*Harrison... *Harrison's review of Internal Medicine*
Kenton, Leslie and Kenton, Susannah: *Endless Energy*. Vermillion Books,
    1993
Kubler Ross, Elizabeth: *On Death and Dying*. Tavistock Publications, 1985
    (first published 1973)
Kubler Ross, Elizabeth: *The Wheel of Life*. Bantam Press, 1997
Mountain Dreamer, *Oriah:The Invitation*. Thorsons, 1999
Mountain Dreamer, *Oriah:The Dance*. Thorsons, 2001
Myss, Caroline: *Anatomy of the Spirit*. Bantam Books, 1997
Noakes, Tim: *Lore of running*. Oxford University Press, 1999
Northrup, C.L: *Women's Bodies, Women's Wisdom*. New York: Bantam
    Books, 1994

Ornish, Dean: *Love and Survival*. London:Vermillion, 1998
Pizzorno J.E and Murray M.T: *Textbook of Natural Medicine 2nd edition*. Churchill-Livingstone, 1999
Rinpoche, Sogyal: *The Tibetan Book of Living and Dying*. Random House, 1992
Schulz, Mona Lisa: *Awakening Intuition*. Bantam Books, 1999
Sears, Barry: *Enter the Zone*. NewYork ReganBooks-Harper Collins, 1995
Siegel, Bernie: *Love, Medicine and Miracles*. Arrow Books, 1988
Weil, Andrew: *Spontaneous Healing*. Warner Books, 1995
Weil, Andrew: *8 Weeks to Optimum Health*. Warner Books, 1997
Weil, Andrew: *Natural Health, Natural Medicine*. Warner Books, 1997

Index